WATER AEROBICS

A. LYNN BERLE

North Carolina State University

KENDALL/HUNT PUBLISHING COMPANY
2460 Kerper Boulevard   P.O. Box 539   Dubuque, Iowa 52004-0539

CONTENTS

PREFACE

The interest in fitness and exercise has increased dramatically in the past few years. People of all ages are walking, jogging, bicycling, swimming, and participating in more aerobic activities than ever before. Regular exercise as a component of wellness is simply a way of life now for much of the population.

Water Aerobics will introduce you to a new, enjoyable, and different way of achieving aerobic fitness. Because you are suspended by the buoyancy of water, the chance of injury from this type of exercise is almost eliminated. Water aerobics is an excellent form of exercise for those with certain medical conditions, such as individuals with knee and/or back problems, cardiac patients, arthritics, and the healthy, young and old alike. Since you do not have to be able to swim to participate, anyone who can stand in chest deep water can enjoy this fun way to exercise.

The first two chapters of this book will review the components of physical fitness and how they relate to total fitness and an aerobic exercise program. Also included, are the general benefits of a healthy, strong body. Establishing individual target heart rates for use in monitoring aerobic exercise will also be explained.

Chapter three will be of particular interest because it deals with the properties of water and how water aerobics differs from regular aerobic exercise or aerobic dance. The additional benefits to be gained by exercising in water will be thoroughly covered, with specific emphasis placed on water resistance and the utilization of resistive equipment.

Chapter four deals with special health and injury questions as they relate to fitness and water aerobics. Special populations such as those persons who may be blind or deaf, or who have muscle, nerve, or bone disorders, will be discussed with ways for adapting the program to fit individual needs. Neither age or the inability to swim should be considered a roadblock to water aerobic participation.

The next three chapters are perhaps the most significant for you as the participant in the program. Specific exercise movements have been designed for use in the water. These are by no means the only exercises you can use. They are simply the base from which you should start your water aerobics program. Variations in movement, formations, and sequence will only help to enhance your interest of an individualized program. Information describing the major muscle groups used in each exercise is included to help move you from your present physical condition to your ultimate fitness goal.

The final chapter assists you in determining your present fitness level. As you become more fit, the intensity, resistance, and duration of the program will increase, and your fitness screening test scores will change.

If there is one concept I would like you to have after developing your water aerobics program, it is that it was not only physically and mentally beneficial, but also fun. In addition to enjoying your water aerobics program, you will be a happier, healthier individual. So, put on your bathing suit, hop in the water, and let's begin!

ACKNOWLEDGMENTS

I would like to extend special thanks to the following people whose help and expertise made this book possible. David C. Falk, Sr. whose financial knowledge provided the means for acquiring a computer for writing this book. Larry Black whose computer knowledge saved me and this manuscript on numerous occasions.

My students—Blair Glass, Steven Doggett, Melinda Dudley, and Mina McKay who rose early on several occasions for the pictures used in this book. Larry Brown who took some of the in water and all of the under water photographs. Lin Ellis whose knowledge and work with special populations was greatly appreciated. Dr. Angela Lumpkin, Donna Clark, Kathy Davis, Jim DeWitt and Ervene Sonner who spent many hours proofreading the manuscript. My parents—Jack and Meriwyn Berle who gave me the gift of an education.

1

Water constitutes nearly 70% or 140,000,000 square miles of the earth's surface. Water provides a living habitat for 9/10 of all plants and animals. Water is the inorganic liquid from which organic liquids are produced, be it the blood in your body or the gas in your car. The human body is more than 75% water. Truly, water is the bearer of life.

Composed of hydrogen and oxygen, this colorless, odorless, transparent liquid is an integral part of everyday living. It keeps you, your clothes,your home, and your car clean. Water provides nourishment for plants and animals and ultimately food for you. Water is the best means of quenching thirst and acts as a cooling agent for your body, food, drink, and many types of machinery. In a gaseous state water can power engines, cook food, and perform other needed functions for society and daily living. The success and happiness you enjoy on earth will, to a large extent, depend on how wisely and how well you utilize this versatile and abundant substance.

Considering the availability of this natural resource, it seems only logical that it be used for recreational purposes. Lakes, rivers, and oceans have been used for years for transportation of goods and people as well as for recreational boating and swimming. With the recent emphasis on fitness and the life-extending benefits of aerobic exercise, swimming and water exercise have grown into popular activities for improving aerobic capacity and overall fitness. If you do not have a natural body of water at your disposal, most communities have public pools. Some of these public pools may already have established water exercise or water aerobic programs.

Why Water Aerobics?

Aerobic dancing first gained popularity in the early 1970s when Jackie Sorenson, who is considered one of the founders of aerobic dance, choreographed hops, skips, jumps, and various arm and leg movements to music. This form of aerobic exercise received wide approval from a health and fitness sensitized public, especially non-joggers. Regular aerobic dance classes became common among scheduled program offerings at many YWCA's and YMCA's, health clubs, city and county recreational facilities, colleges, and universities. As the popularity of this type of exercise increased, new forms and names were introduced, such as Jazzercise, Dancercise, and Aerobicise.

Along with the increase in the number of classes being offered and an increase in participation, came a growing problem with injuries. The strain placed on the body's lower extremities from the jumping, hopping, and kicking motions caused considerable hip, knee, shin, ankle, and foot problems, especially for the beginner or more sedentary participant. Due to the increase in injuries resulting from aerobic dance exercises, participants began to drop out of these programs and question the long-term benefits of a form of exercise that produced such injuries. In order to eliminate the drop in participation and frequent injury problems, low-impact aerobics was introduced.

Low-impact aerobics is a form of exercise which utilizes large arm movements, but eliminates jumping and hopping, replacing these movements with leg and foot motions low to the ground. The major difference between aerobic dance and low-impact aerobics is one foot is on the ground at all times during a low-impact workout. By keeping one foot in contact with the floor at all times, jarring of the lower extremities that accompanied original aerobic dance workouts is greatly reduced.

Water aerobics goes one step beyond low-impact aerobics. As Diane Grimes and Joseph Krasevec stress in their book *HydroRobics*, two key properties of water buoyancy and resistance—make water exercise a non-weight bearing, strength and endurance building form of exercise. The resistance of the water helps achieve or maintain fitness through the use of vigorous underwater movements over a specific period of time, while the non-weight bearing, or buoyancy property of water prevents the jerky, jarring motions common to traditional aerobics. This type of exercise places considerably less strain on the limbs and joints. Water aerobics eliminates previous injury problems related to aerobic dance and other high-impact aerobic programs.

Water aerobics can be described as the use of specific exercises, that have been adapted for use in the water, for the purpose of maintaining or increasing cardiovascular endurance, muscular strength and endurance, and flexibility. Specific exercise movements involving large muscle groups of the arms and legs are choreographed by the instructor and set to music. Since all movements are performed in shallow water, the ability to swim is not a requirement for participation, although it is strongly recommended. Many non-swimmers find this form of exercise an ideal lead-up activity to becoming more comfortable in the water and ultimately in learning how to swim.

Benefits of Water Aerobics

There are certain exercise benefits derived from participation in a water aerobics program that are not experienced in other exercise programs. The benefits you enjoy during, or as a result of any exercise program, are directly related to your dedication, enthusiasm, effort, and willingness to work hard for total fitness. When you exercise on land you do not experience a noticeable degree of air resistance, but when you exercise in water, the resistance causes you to expend more energy to complete a motion. Due to this resistance provided by pushing, pulling, or lifting the water, you can gain improved fitness. The buoyancy provided by the water also tends to change sudden, jerky movements into predictably smoother motions. The possibility of muscle injuries such as sprains or strains, is greatly decreased. Since you are immersed in water from the chest down, you can exercise both upper and lower body parts against resistance simultaneously. This has the overall effect of toning the midsection of the body more efficiently than any other aerobic exercise.

Most exercise machines work specific muscle groups against the pull of gravity, isolating not only the muscle but limiting the direction of movement. Water is a three-dimensional resistance medium. The arms and/or legs can be moved in any direction with equal resistance. This provides for an equal amount of work being done by opposing muscle groups. Normally, you would have to do one set of exercises for the quadriceps (front of thigh) and one set for the hamstrings (back of thigh); in the water one exercise can work both muscle groups equally and simultaneously.

The density of water not only provides increased resistance, but also produces the buoyancy effect. The support given to the body by the property of buoyancy is the closest thing to weightlessness that you will probably ever experience. For this reason, water aerobics is an excellent form of exercise if you have joint-related injury problems. The trauma and stress to the joints from dry-land activities are eliminated due to the supportive buoyancy of water, which provides needed support to the spine, hips, and knees, and allows the joints to move through a full range of motion.

If you have ever put water in a pan and added melted butter or oil to it, you will find that fat floats! Fat in the body does the same thing in water it floats. Therefore, water aerobics is an excellent form of exercise for those who are overweight, because it makes them feel much lighter and reduces the amount of discomfort and self-consciousness that may accompany being overweight. The weightlessness of the body in water decreases joint, ligament, and muscle problems frequently experienced by the overweight individual during dry-land aerobic exercise programs. Furthermore, many people who are obese cannot not safely participate in a dry-land aerobic program, but are able to experience a good, safe, and productive exercise workout with water aerobic exercises.

From a physiological viewpoint, muscle activity or exercises done in water, rather than in air, will put less strain on the heart and circulatory system. Equal levels of large muscle activity done in the water requires fewer beats of the heart per minute. For this reason, you can gain more muscle toning with the same heart rate in water aerobics than from other dynamic aerobic activities.

Heart rate during exercise is also affected by temperature. Immersion in cool water will automatically lower the pulse. The water temperature in most pools is kept around 80 degrees fahrenheit. This has the effect of decreasing the pulse 5–10 beats per minute. Since the heart does not have to work as hard to cool the body, less blood is sent to the skin for cooling purposes and more blood goes to the working muscles, increasing the efficiency of the circulatory system.

This cooling effect of water allows the body to lose heat twice as fast as in the air. One reason for this is that the greater surface area available for heat transfer disperses the body heat to the surrounding water. If the water is warm, you may exercise at a slower pace and still achieve your exercise or target heart rate since more blood is needed to cool the body. Even with the cooling of the water, perspiration does occur, but general overheating of the body is prevented with water aerobics.

Making Exercise Fun

Exercise is a wonderful outlet to help you relax, feel better, and eliminate or cope with stress, and most importantly it is fun! Participation in water aerobics usually involves a group of people with similar interests and goals toward exercise. You may be interested in increasing your fitness level, controlling your appetite and/or body weight, toning muscles and body shape, or participating in a new and different exercise program ''just for the fun of it!'' Water aerobics is ideal for all these reasons. Since you are in chest high water, you do not even have to worry about getting your head wet. The attitude you bring to class will determine to a great degree the fitness benefits obtained from the water aerobics class and the amount of fun you have while participating. You will be helping yourself mentally and physically while you are exercising, because water aerobics will help your heart and cir culatory system. You are decreasing your chance for heart disease and may even be lengthening your life.

PHYSICAL FITNESS AND WATER AEROBICS

2

Physical fitness is frequently defined as the ability to perform normal, daily activities without undue fatigue and still have reserve energy to handle emergency situations. Normal, daily activities may include a job, family or civic duties, club meetings and recreational pursuits as well as any number of other activities encountered in the busy, mobile society of today. In the past, physical fitness was not considered a necessity to a healthy way of life since much of the work performed was manual and naturally required a certain degree of fitness. In today's technically oriented society, more time is spent sitting at a desk, striking a computer keyboard, pushing buttons, driving a car, or sitting in front of the television set than in active physical labor. Recent studies, conducted by exercise physiologists, have made us aware of our lack of conditioning and created renewed interest in the significance of general wellness and good physical fitness so that we may live a happier, healthier, and more prosperous lifestyle. The concepts of wellness and physical fitness need to be integrated into daily living and practiced by all of society.

Participation in a specific sport in which you are reasonably skilled, does not necessarily mean you are also physically fit. To be considered physically fit you must meet all the criteria for cardiovascular endurance, muscular strength and endurance, and flexibility. For instance, if you participate in a regular weight lifting program, you may fulfill the fitness requirements of muscular strength and muscular endurance; but, unless you are also engaging in aerobic and flexibility activities you will not be considered physically fit. Often an athlete will meet one or two of the fitness components, but *all* of the criteria must be fulfilled to become totally fit.

Water aerobics offers an excellent form of activity that will meet all of the fitness criteria. Because of the resistance provided by working in the water, contributions are made to all four components of fitness. Jogging satisfies the component of aerobic or cardiovascular endurance. Resistive equipment and the natural resistance of the water fulfills the requirements for good muscular strength and muscular endurance. The warm-up and cooldown for each of these activities includes flexibility work. You cannot achieve total fitness through participation in only one of these activities.

Components of Physical Fitness

As stated above, there are four basic components of physical fitness. Some fitness specialists include a fifth—body composition as a measurement of total fitness. Since water aerobics provides a less stressful training situation for altering body composition, this factor will be included in the discussion that follows.

Cardiovascular endurance is the ability of the heart, lungs, and circulatory system to carry oxygen and nutrients to the muscles and to remove waste products. Cardiovascular endurance is achieved through participation in an appropriate aerobic activity as opposed to an anaerobic activity. Activities that involve spurts of power in a start and stop manner are considered anaerobic. Tennis, especially doubles, would be considered an anaerobic activity. Anaerobic means ''without air''. In essence you are borrowing oxygen from the body and replacing it later by placing the cardiovascular system into oxygen debt. Anaerobic activity does not depend on the air you are breathing during exercise since the duration of the activity is usually less than one minute. For this reason, anaerobic exercise does not meet the criteria for improving cardiovascular endurance.

Aerobic means ''with air'' or utilizing oxygen. Aerobic exercise requires large amounts of oxygen transfer during activity over an extended period of time. When an activity is done on a regular basis for an extended time period, it will improve the heart's pumping ability as well as the circulatory system's ability to transport oxygen more efficiently. Oxygen is inhaled into the lungs where it is diffused into the blood and carried mostly by the red blood cells to the working muscles and other body parts. During aerobic exercise, a balance is reached between the intake and expenditure of oxygen. This improves the body's ability to process oxygen effectively, resulting in an improvement in aerobic capacity and cardiovascular endurance.

Guidelines for Developing Cardiovascular Endurance

Exercise Style

To achieve cardiovascular benefit through exercise, an activity must involve large muscle usage over an extended period of time and be continuous in nature. Activities such as jogging, running, aerobic dance, water aerobics, swimming, rope skipping, and bicycling are considered excellent activities for improving aerobic capacity.

Frequency

In order to provide functional benefit to the heart, lungs, and circulatory system, an aerobic activity must be done 3 to 5 days per week. Three days a week will maintain your present fitness level, while fewer days of participation will show a decrease in aerobic capacity.

Intensity

Heart rate monitoring during participation in aerobic activity is the most efficient means of ensuring an aerobic benefit from exercise. You must exercise from 60%–90% of your predicted maximum heart rate for cardiovascular improvement. Heart rate monitoring will be discussed later in this chapter (see page 00).

Duration

It is recommended that 20–60 minutes of actual aerobic exercise be performed for appropriate aerobic benefit. Cardiovascular endurance requires that the activity must be continuous in nature and utilize oxygen directly for energy: exercising for a sustained length of time is vital to your goal of total fitness.

Muscular strength is the maximum amount of force exerted against immediate resistance develops muscular strength. For example, you pick up the end of a sofa and than put it back down. The action was immediate and required a maximum amount of force. Lack of muscular strength produces loose, sagging, flabby muscles. One of the major causes of low back pain is weak abdominal muscles. Improving your muscular strength is another benefit of exercising with water resistance.

Guidelines for Developing Muscular Strength

Exercise Style

The most common means of achieving muscular strength is through a basic weight training program that concentrates on isolating and using specific muscle groups. This can be accomplished in water aerobics by adding resistive equipment, such as hand paddles, to be used with specific exercises designed to strengthen specific muscles or muscle groups.

Frequency

Use of weights should be limited to 3 days per week or every other day depending on your workout schedule. In water aerobics, once a good level of strength is achieved, resistive equipment can be used more frequently. The possibility of overworking the muscle or muscle groups to the point of injury is decreased due to the buoyancy of the water.

Intensity

To gain absolute strength, weight work should include more resistance (heavier weights, larger hand paddles) and fewer repetitions. Multiple wrist and/or ankle weights can be worn to increase resistance.

Duration

The time required to complete 2–3 sets of an exercise will vary. You should try to isolate a specific muscle or muscle group for greatest improvement and strength gain.

Muscular endurance is the amount of force a muscle or group of muscles can exert over an extended period of time. For example, you pick up the end of a sofa. Hold the sofa in an elevated position for a period of time, then lower it to the floor. When dealing with muscular strength or muscular endurance, the differentiating factor is time. It is important to note that muscular endurance is a prerequisite to cardiovascular endurance.

Guidelines for Developing Muscular Endurance

Exercise Style

Exercises that are calisthenic in nature are used most frequently to achieve muscular endurance. In water aerobics, no wrist or ankle weights need to be used for endurance work initially since the medium of water itself acts as resistance.

Frequency

To gain endurance, muscular activity should be done 3–5 days per week. This is consistent with the frequency of participation required for cardiovascular endurance. With both endurance factors, the continuous, extended nature of an exercise is essential.

Intensity

To increase dynamic endurance, you should use less resistance and more repetitions. In water aerobics, the water will provide initial and continuous resistance and the number of times you execute the exercise will be increased.

Duration

The time required to complete 2–3 sets of a specific exercise will vary according to your strength and endurance.

Flexibility is the ability of a joint to move through a full range of motion. With age, the degree of flexibility within a specific joint will decrease. The greater the amount of flexibility in a joint, the less chance there is of injury to the joint and surrounding tissue. The degree of flexibility in a joint will vary according to the shape of the bone and cartilage, and the length of the muscle and ligaments that are specific to the joint.

Guidelines for Developing Flexibility

Exercise Style

Passive exercises or static stretching exercises are those in which the muscle is slowly stretched to the point of tension and held there for a set period of time, concentrating on specific muscle groups. Active or ballistic stretching involves bouncing or jerking into the exercise and may cause overstretching of the muscles and/or tendons. This can be dangerous and result in serious injury. Stretching should always be passive to avoid possible injury.

Frequency

Flexibility or stretching exercises should be done prior to any exercise period or workout and also be included in the cool down. It is recommended that flexibility exercises be done a minimum of 3 days per week to decrease the chance of muscle and joint injuries.

Intensity

The execution of the specific stretching exercise should require you to move through the full range of motion (active stretch) and hold the stretch when tension of the muscle is felt (passive stretch).

Duration

It is recommended that 10–20 repetitions of an exercise for each specific muscle group be done, with tension held for 10–20 seconds. The time factor in most exercise programs will usually limit specific exercise repetitions to 3–5, held for 6–10 seconds. This is not ideal, but will usually provide sufficient muscle stretch prior to, and following exercise to eliminate the chance of injury.

Body composition is the percentage of body fat compared to your lean body mass, which includes both muscle and bone. The best and most accurate method for determining lean body mass is through submersion in water. Since fat floats, a low percentage of body fat will cause you to weigh more in water due to the fact that lean body mass is heavier than fat. Few programs or facilities have a water tank for this hydrostatic weighing, so percent body fat is determined through skinfold measurements using a set of skinfold calipers.

Exercise physiologists have found that the average percent body fat for an adult male is 15–19% of his body weight and for an adult female 18–22% of her body weight. Excess fat that causes you to exceed these percentages can lead to obesity. Being overweight or overfat can place additional stress on the cardiovascular system, as well as the joints, and is a serious health risk. It is estimated that up to 50% of the U.S. population is considered overweight or obese and unless our eating habits change drastically, this figure may increase in the future.

Heart Rate Monitoring

In the United States alone, over 66% of the deaths due to heart attacks are related to poor cardiovascular efficiency and another 20% of strokes are caused by cardiovascular disease. The heart is a muscle and an extremely important one! However, it ages and wears out. The heart can be trained to work more efficiently, causing it to last longer by pumping the same amount of blood in fewer beats. This is the main reason it is important to participate in an aerobic activity that builds and maintains cardiovascular endurance.

Checking your heart rate is the easiest and most practical means of estimating aerobic output. As you exercise, the body's need for oxygen increases, so the heart must pump more blood. This causes the heart to beat faster and to work harder. Your heart rate acts as a measuring device for the frequency at which the heart is pumping, hence a larger volume of blood is being circulated.

Your heart rate can be most easily taken at two pulse sites: the radial artery and the carotid artery. The radial artery is located at the wrist bone on the thumb side of the hand. The radial pulse should always be taken with the first and second fingers of the opposite hand. Do not try to take the radial pulse with the thumb. The thumb has a pulse, making it almost impossible to feel the radial pulse and to take an accurate count.

The carotid pulse is located beside the esophagus in the neck. Place the two middle fingers of the hand on the back of the mandible (jaw bone) and slide the fingers forward on the neck. Be sure not to apply too much pressure. Pressure on this area of the neck will not only slow the pulse rate, but it will also slow the flow of blood to the head.

To establish your resting heart rate (RHR), take your pulse on 2–3 consecutive mornings before getting out of bed. If possible, take it for one full minute to achieve the most accurate count. If you are unable to keep count for a full minute, take a 30 second count and multiply by 2 or take a 15 second count and multiply by 4. Remember, the longer you count up to one minute, the more accurate your resting heart rate.

During exercise, rather than taking the pulse count for 30–60 seconds, take your pulse count for 6 seconds and multiply by 10 to attain your one-minute rate or take your pulse rate for 10 seconds and multiply by 6 to attain your one-minute pulse rate. The taking of your exercise pulse should not allow the heart rate to drop or interrupt the continuous exercise period.

Maximum heart rate (MHR) is considered the highest heart rate taken at the point of exhaustion after exercise. In the 1950's, Astrand established a formula to best estimate your maximum heart rate attainable upon exhaustion. Take the constant number of 220bpm (beats per minute) and from this subtract your age. For example, if you are 19 years old, take 220–19=201 or a maximum heart rate of 201bpm.

Now that you are able to find your pulse and take your resting heart rate, you can establish a means for determining the intensity level of your aerobic workout. Your target heart rate (THR) is the upper and lower heart rate level you must achieve during exercise to gain an aerobic benefit from the exercise period.

There are several methods used to establish target heart rate. The most accurate is the formula developed by Karvonen in the 1960's. His formula considers not only your maximum heart rate but also your resting heart rate. The Karvonen formula for establishing target heart rate is:

$$60\% \text{ or } 90\% \text{ (MHR–RHR)} + \text{RHR} = \text{Target Heart Rate(THR)}$$

If you use the maximum heart rate of 201 that was established earlier for a 19-year old, and a resting pulse of 68 bpm, to find 60% or the lower target heart rate you take:

$$60\% \text{ or } .60(201–68)+68=147.8 \text{ lower THR}$$

To determine 90% or the upper target heart rate you take:

$$90\% \text{ or} .90(201–68)+68=187.7 \text{ upper THR}$$

The aerobic workout should keep your heart rate at or within the lower and upper target heart rates established by the Karvonen formula. If your heart rate is below 60% THR, you are not working hard enough to gain any aerobic benefit from the exercise. Likewise, if your pulse is above 90% THR, you are working too hard and are getting into a danger zone. Increase or decrease your intensity appropriately. Monitor your heart rate periodically during exercise to make sure you are within your lower and upper THR for aerobic benefit.

Immediately following an aerobic workout, your pulse should be checked. At the end of one minute, take your pulse again to establish your recovery rate. This period of one minute is considered part of the cool-down and is also considered the pulse recovery rate. The faster the heart returns to your resting pulse rate, the better condition you are in aerobically. As your aerobic capacity increases, your heart will require less time to return to a resting rate. This is an indication that the heart, lungs and circulatory system are functioning more efficiently.

There are some specific factors that have a significant influence on your heart rate. These factors help explain the variance you may find not only in your own heart rate at different times, but also in your heart rate compared to other individuals, especially your peer group. Some of the major influences and the effect they have on the heart rate are:

1. Age—decreases maximum heart rate
2. Caffeine—increases heart rate
3. Exercise—decreases resting heart rate
4. Food digestion—increases resting heart rate
5. Medication—increases heart rate
6. Pregnancy—increases heart rate
7. Sex—females heart rate is 5–10 bpm higher than males
8. Smoking—increases heart rate
9. Stress—increases heart rate
10. Temperature—hot/humid weather increases heart rate 10–40 bpm

11. Weight gain—increases heart rate

The only factor on this list that will decrease your heart rate and which you can control is exercise.

Improving Physical Fitness

Everyone begins an exercise program at a different fitness level. Most people entering an exercise routine have an ultimate goal such as weight control, improving body image, muscle toning, or an increased level of fitness. To improve your fitness level, you must apply what is referred to as the "overload principle" to your exercise program. This simply means making specific muscle groups work harder by overloading them, thus increasing the strength and efficiency of the muscles. Overload can be achieved by varying the frequency, intensity, and/or duration of the activity.

Frequency overload may involve an increase in the number of workouts per week. This can be easily experienced when dealing with cardiovascular endurance. Studies have shown that cardiovascular improvement is directly proportional to the amount of overload or additional stress placed on the heart, lungs, and circulatory system.

Intensity can also be applied to the overload principle. By increasing the number of repetitions done when exercising a specific muscle group, muscular endurance can be improved. In addition, many exercises can be adapted to increase the amount of resistance and degree of difficulty. The increased difficulty of the exercise will strengthen and improve the function of specific muscle groups. In water aerobics, adding resistive equipment such as hand paddles, ankle and wrist weights, arm fins and/or power wings, will overload the muscles resulting in more work being done against the force of the water.

Of course, the duration and/or time spent performing the exercises can be varied. As your fitness level improves, you will want to lengthen your aerobic workouts. This will gradually increase your fitness level. The improvement will be evident in a faster pulse drop during the recovery period. Ultimately, your target heart rate will need adjusting as your resting pulse decreases due to increased aerobic capacity.

Additional stress can be placed on the system by increasing the tempo or speed of the music and exercises. Increasing the length of the workout and the speed of the workout should not be done simultaneously. This may place too much overload on the system and lead to fatigue, soreness, and injury problems. Heart rate monitoring and "listening" to your body are the best measuring devices for determining appropriate overload.

Benefits of Exercise

The benefits derived from regular exercise extend well beyond the components of physical fitness. Listed below are some of the most recognizable benefits derived from a regular exercise program.

1. Exercise tends to curb the appetite for 2–3 hours following activity.

2. Exercise tends to elevate the body's basal metabolism, thus burning more calories and aiding in weight control.

3. Exercise tends to increase HDL (high density lipoprotein), or good cholesterol, and decrease LDL (low density lipoprotein), or bad cholesterol in the body.

4. Exercise helps control the physical and emotional stress, tension, and fatigue of everyday living.

5. Exercise tends to improve your intellectual capacity and increases productivity.

6. Exercise and physical fitness are significant factors in protecting your body from heart disease.

7. Exercise and physical fitness will make the heart muscle stronger and increase lung capacity.

8. Exercise makes bones stronger and thicker.

9. Exercise will help improve your self-concept.

10. Exercise will increase your energy level.

11. Exercise will enable you to sleep better and to feel more rested in the morning.

12. Exercise will provide an opportunity for you to meet new people and make new friends.

13. Exercise is good for young and old alike. There is no age barrier when it comes to looking and feeling good.

Your body must support and carry you through a lifetime of daily activity. It seems only fair that you provide your body with the proper care so it can function at optimal capacity. To accomplish this, the body needs not only food and rest, but regular exercise. These benefits are major contributors to the sudden increase in social awareness of the importance of exercise.

In water aerobics, the benefits you derive from the workout depends upon the amount of force you exert. The larger the area of water that is pulled or pushed, the greater the benefit. For best results, motions of the arms and legs should be exaggerated in the water and moved through the full range of motion, thus producing the greatest amount of water resistance. You can feel the water being pushed away from your body or pulled toward your body. Often the range of motion of the arms or legs is increased in water aerobics, due to the buoyancy. Each muscle, or group of muscles, is actually forced to work harder in the water because of the additional water resistance when pushing or pulling motions are performed. The harder you push, the harder the water pushes back.

Exercise motions performed in the water will automatically be slowed because of water resistance. When additional resistive equipment is added to the exercise, the difficulty of the exercise is increased and the speed of the exercise will again decrease. For these reasons, it is important to keep the pace of the exercise moving. If the speed of the exercise is slowed too much, the force is lowered and the workout's efficiency decreases. Therefore, maintain the speed of the exercise at a reasonably brisk pace for greatest water resistance and benefit. This is especially important when jogging in the water and/or executing wide-arm movements. When jogging, the quadriceps should push the water forcefully toward the surface of the pool.

To achieve the greatest degree of muscular, as well as cardiovascular benefits from water exercise, the motions should be forceful and brisk. Slow, flowing, melodic motions will massage the muscles, but they will not develop the strength, endurance, and toning effect to their optimum.

Properties of Water

The five basic properties of water are: resistance, buoyancy, temperature, pressure, and massage. All of these affect your exercise program. How the body responds to exercise in the water will be directly proportional to the effort you expend. Some will have a greater physiological affect on the system than others, but all properties work to the betterment of the total human being.

Resistance

The single most important property of water for improving the quality of the muscles both in strength and endurance is resistance. As stated earlier, water resistance supports the exercise principle of overload thus increasing the efficiency of the muscles. The resistance of the water can be adapted to increase muscular strength and/or muscular endurance. Water is not gravity-dependent, so the resistance allows you to work both halves of a pair of muscles at the same time and at an equal level of force. The faster the exercise movement in the water, the heavier the resistance will feel. Besides building muscular strength and endurance, the constant resistance provided by water will improve muscle tone and blood circulation and encourage deeper breathing.

Buoyancy

Archimedes' law of physics states that a body immersed in a fluid is buoyed up by the force equal to the weight of the fluid the body displaces. In simple terms, the buoyancy of the water helps support the body, decreasing the chance of injury during exercise and permitting the movement to be more comfortable and sometimes easier. This can be a major factor when deciding how to begin or how to continue an exercise program especially if you are overweight, have joint or muscle problems, or other specific medical restrictions. The water's natural buoyancy will prevent the jerky, pounding motions prevalent in some land workouts thus eliminating most chances of injury and making exercise in the water a more relaxing and pleasant experience.

Temperature

The average temperature of the human body is 98.6 degrees F. Most indoor pools are kept from 83 degrees F–86 degrees F and outdoor pools from 78 degrees F–84 degrees F. Ideal water temperature for exercise is 80 degrees F. This temperature allows the body to eliminate excess heat produced through exercise and to maintain a normal body temperature. Exercise should never be performed in a hot tub or jacuzzi since temperatures can reach as high as 110 degrees F. Water temperatures this high can decrease blood volume resulting in fainting and can raise the body's temperature enough to create an imbalance in the biochemical system.

Warm water, not hot water, produces some beneficial effects to the muscular system. We know that during the warm-up period the blood flow to the muscles is increased; thereby, raising the heat in the muscles and increasing elasticity. When the body is surrounded by warm water during the warm up exercises, the muscle elasticity increases at a faster rate. In addition, the chance of incurring a muscle-related injury is reduced greatly if not eliminated totally. The warming effect of the water will also increase the range of motion for the joints since the muscles and tendons are more elastic. A slower exercise pace can be used in warm water because the pulse will reach the target area sooner.

In cool water, more blood is dispersed to the working muscles so the efficiency of the circulatory system is increased. When the water temperature is in the upper 70's to low 80's, your pulse will normally decrease as much a 5–10 bpm. This is due to the heat lost from your body through the water, consequently, less blood is needed at the surface of the skin to keep it cool. It is estimated that the body will lose heat about twice as fast in the water as on land because there is a greater surface area available for heat transfer.

Some researchers and exercise physiologists are questioning the cardiovascular benefits of water aerobics. They feel the cooling affect of the water on your body results in a lower heart rate. If the intensity of the water aerobics program is challenging enough to the cardiovascular system and the resistance property of water is utilized to the optimum, then an increase in cardiorespiratory endurance can be realized. Proper instruction and exercise intensity will ensure the development of this fitness component.

Pressure

Gravity places a specific amount of pressure on the body. Whether on land or in the water, pressure is evident. It is estimated that water pressure per square inch on the body is greater than the 14.7 pounds per square inch of pressure the body sustains on land. This increased pressure has two effects on the body: 1) pressure tends to stimulate the circulation of the blood through the system; and 2) pressure also causes the respiratory system to work harder. Certain populations, especially those who feel uncomfortable in water, can actually feel the sensation of water pressing against the chest and rib cage. Most people, however, will not even realize the pressure of the water on the system.

Massage

The most relaxing property of water is its massaging effect, created by the water pressure and resistance as the body moves through the water. The warmer the water is, the stronger the massage, because skin circulation is increased. This is the general feeling you will get from hot tubs and jacuzzi's. The "massage effect" is not promoted as a benefit of water aerobics, but it has significant merit for those with medical problems who may require extensive therapeutic and rehabilitative programs.

Resistive Equipment

The popularity of water aerobics as a highly desirable form of fitness exercise, has helped promote the development of new and different equipment for use in water exercise programs. New equipment is being introduced at a rapid pace, providing a greater selection from which to choose. There is some equipment available at local sport retail shops that can be adapted for use in water aerobic programs. A few examples of the resistive equipment that can be used are described below.

Hand Paddles

Hand paddles are used extensively by swimming programs and swim teams to increase arm strength, stroke efficiency, and endurance. Paddles come in various sizes. The hand paddles pictured below range from small in size (4″ x 7″), to medium (4 5/8″ x 7 5/8″), to large (5 1/4″ x 8″). As your strength and endurance improves, you can increase your overload to the selected muscle group by adding hand paddles first, and then later increasing the size of the paddles.

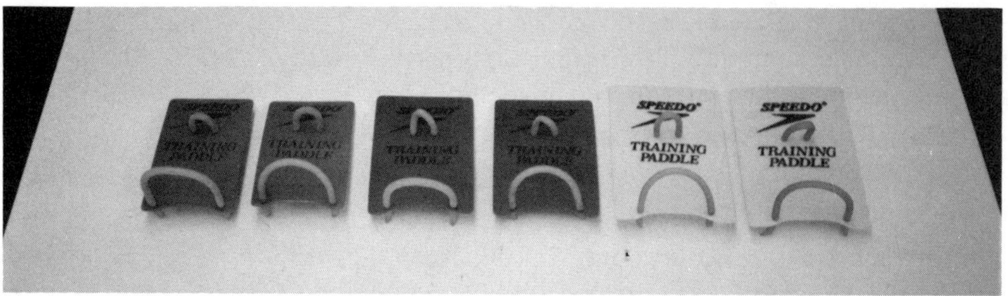

Shoes

Resistance to the lower extremities can be increased by wearing a pair of shoes while exercising in the water. A pair of old tennis shoes, jogging, or aerobic shoes will do nicely. Canvas or nylon shoes are better to wear in the water than leather because they hold up longer and dry more quickly. Make sure the shoes are clean of all dirt, sand and debris. Do not tie a knot in the laces or you may have difficulty removing the shoes at the conclusion of the water aerobics class since fabric laces swell in water. Shoes that have been used for water aerobics should be used only for this purpose. If the additional resistance provided by the shoe causes pain or discomfort to the shins, knees or back, discontinue use immediately.

Flugels

Flugels were designed to help the non-swimmer by increasing buoyancy because the water resistance experienced during exercise is increased. The flugels are inflated causing you to float and decreasing exercise impact to nothing.

Wrist and Ankle Weights

Wrist and ankle weights have been used in aerobic dance and low-impact aerobic programs for quite some time. Some have been used for water aerobics but problems have

Printed with permission of Adolph Kiefer and Associates, 1750 Harding Road, Northfield, IL 60202.
Printed with permission of Speedo America.

occurred with the material used, size of the weight, and weight clasps. New, improved wrist and ankle weights are being introduced for use in water aerobics. The two sets of weights pictured below were designed for use in water aerobics and weigh 1 to 2 1/4 pounds each. The wider pair were designed for ankle use and weigh 2 1/4 pounds each. The lighter weights can be used on either the wrists or ankles and weigh 1 pound each.

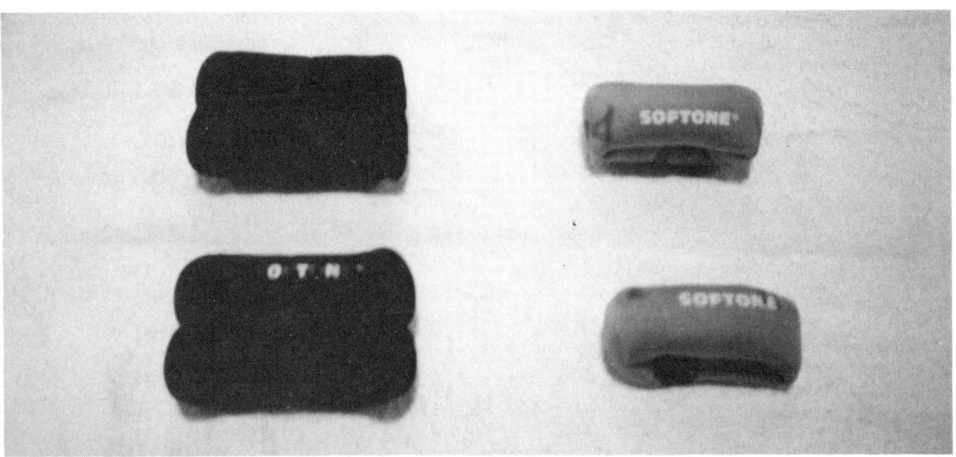

Wet Vest

A 2-pound device made of neoprene and Lycra, called a wet vest, enables a person lacking natural buoyancy to float upright in deep water. It eliminates the necessity to expend energy for the sole purpose of staying up in the water. The wet vest allows a non-buoyant person to concentrate on the exercise being performed and the resistance being applied rather than on staying afloat.

Power Wings

Power wings are placed on the forearm to add resistance to the upper body. They consist of a cuff placed around the forearm to eliminate any irritation from the wing apparatus. The wing consists of two hinged plastic scoops designed to fit on either side of the forearm and to open and close as the arm is pulled through the water. Velcro straps allow the wings to be adjusted for various arm sizes. The wings should be snug on the cuff to hinder sliding of the wing up and down or around the arm. Be sure the cuff and/or wing are not too tight

Printed with permission of Durward Industries, LTD, 11-564 Weber Street N., Waterloo, Ontario, Canada N2L5C6

causing discomfort to the arm or numbness in the hand and fingers. The photo below shows the cuffs on the left side of the picture and the wings on the right side.

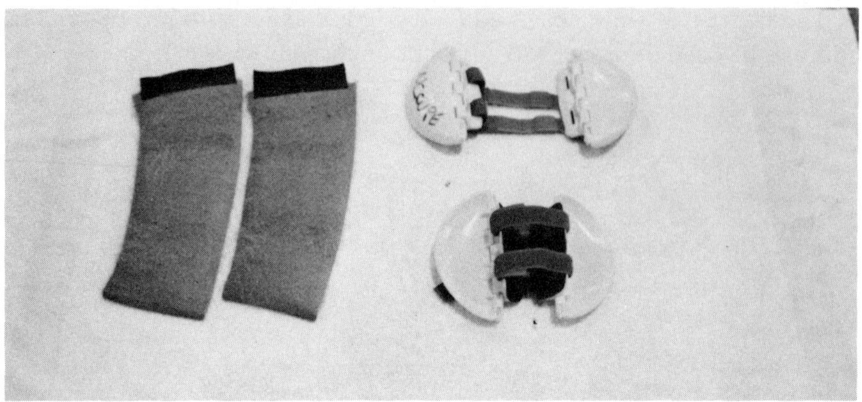

Therapeutic Benefits

Water exercise has definite therapeutic benefits for those persons who cannot participate in regular exercise programs due to injury and for those who are in medically-designed and monitored hydrotherapy programs. Perhaps the greatest therapeutic benefit of water aerobics is the fact that water exercise is fun and relaxing. In the stressful society of today, any activity that allows for fitness benefit and relaxation is sure to improve your attitude and productivity.

Water buoyancy helps with individual injury problems such as shin splints and muscle strains. Exercises can be modified so that participation can continue even after certain injuries occur. Many athletic trainers and coaches have included water exercises in their injured athletes' exercise programs. Water aerobics seems to eliminate the frustration some athletes feel due to inactivity during recovery from an injury. Similar movements related to a specific sport can be adapted for use in the pool aiding the athlete not only physically, but psychologically.

Experts agree that the soothing, massaging nature of water exercise helps to relax the muscles and acts as a distraction from the frequent pain of recovery. The healing time required for most knee and arm injuries decreases due to water exercise workouts. Caution should be taken when using water exercises for therapeutic purposes. Water that is too warm or too cold can increase the pain to someone experiencing a serious muscle spasm.

SAFETY CONSIDERATIONS 4

When starting any exercise program there are certain aspects to consider for good, safe exercise. Water aerobics presents some additional safety precautions due to the nature of the medium in which you are exercising. Some basic exercise guidelines to follow for a safe water aerobics program are listed below.

1. Always work with a partner.
2. Glasses should be stabilized by the use of a guard strap.
3. Goggles may be worn with contact lenses if preferred.
4. Entrance into the water should be gradual.
5. During the exercises breathe evenly, rhythmically, and deeply.
6. All stretching should be of a static nature slow and steady.
7. Always warm-up properly before exercising and cool-down following the exercise period.
8. Never chew gum or eat while participating in a water aerobic program.
9. Never eat a meal just prior to participating in a water aerobics program.
10. Women should wear bathing suits that provide good support for the breasts.
11. If you are not accustomed to regular exercise, pregnant, a "weekend athlete," or over 35 years of age, check with your doctor before starting a water aerobics program.

Pregnancy

Pregnancy should not be a condition that will eliminate exercise for most females. Although certain adjustments need to be made in your exercise program during pregnancy, participation can continue up to the onset of labor. Water aerobics and the affect it has on the heart and lungs will help to deal with the breathing patterns required during delivery. However, if you have not been participating in a regular exercise program prior to pregnancy, make sure you check with a physician before starting a program.

Water aerobics may be better for women during pregnancy than any other form of exercise. It is less stressful on the mother's body than exercising on land because of the buoying effect of the water and the non-weight bearing support of the water. The elimination of the pull of gravity relieves abdominal pressure and discomfort frequently experienced during pregnancy. In addition, by utilizing exercises that strengthen the abdominal muscles, it can help eliminate low back pain that can accompany the additional weight placement of the fetus.

Water aerobics will also reduce the thermal stress felt during pregnancy by lowering the mother's body temperature. For this to occur, the water must be cool since warm water will have just the opposite effect on the circulatory system causing the mother's body temperature to rise.

Special Populations

Water aerobics can serve as a great form of exercise for those who have specific health or medical limitations. This includes medical conditions that develop due to accidents, sickness, heredity, and birth. In most cases, what some people consider physical limitations to exercise participation can be dealt with through adaptations of the exercises to meet their needs. The water provides an exercise medium for a number of people to whom exercise is either extremely difficult or impossible.

Visual Impairments

Visual impairments are best classified according to the degree of functional loss in depth perception, muscular action of the eyes or peripheral vision. A person is considered to be visually impaired if they measure below 20/20 on the Sneller Scale. A person is classified legally blind if their corrected vision is 20/200 or less. Partial or total vision loss can usually be attributed to infection, injury, or some congenital defect.

To aid the visually impaired during participation in a water aerobics program, it is important to make sure the individual is given the opportunity to fully explore and familiarize themselves with the environment both on land and in the pool. Any barriers such as steps, walls, furniture, and water depth should be fully explored before the start of the program. Outside noises or other disturbances should be removed or at least minimized as much as possible.

Water aerobics provides an excellent medium for physical fitness development for the visually impaired. As long as certain precautions are followed, the program can progress with very little exercise adaptations. Here are some things to consider when working with an individual that is visually impaired.

1. Always make sure the ''buddy system'' is adhered to strictly.
2. Use clear and concise tactile and auditory cues.
3. Remove or minimize all hazards or barriers.
4. Keep the head above water due to the importance of auditory cuing.

5. Be aware of the problems the visually impaired have with depth perception and balance.

6. Guide the visually impaired through specific exercise movements tactually at first.

Orthopaedic Impairment

Orthopaedic impairments are disorders of the bones, joints, tendons, blood vessels, and nerves that impede locomotor functions. They can range in degree of restrictions from short- term sprains or strains to the permanent loss of a limb or limbs. Orthopaedic impairments are usually caused by injury, trauma, congenital condition and infection.

Depending upon the degree of impairment, sensory responses in the extremities may be low or absent leaving open the possibility for scrapes and abrasions. Caution should be taken when exercising at the side of the pool to avoid hitting the side or bottom of the pool structure. Poor circulation may also accompany this disorder making the onset of fatigue and chilling more prevalent. More time should be allocated for rest periods and water adjustment to maintain reasonable exercise comfort. Amputees may be more buoyant and require resistive equipment to achieve their balance.

The benefits of a water aerobics program for the orthopaedically impaired are social, emotional, and physical in scope. The individual can acquire lasting benefits from these exercises in the following areas:

1. Improved muscle tone and stronger postural muscles.

2. Improved breathing through the increase in cardiovascular efficiency and strengthening of the breathing muscles.

3. Improved ambulation when unable to achieve this on land.

4. Increased circulation, healing, and relief of constant pressure on areas that are susceptible to skin breakdown.

5. Improved self-esteem.

6. Freedom from assistance devices.

7. Increased functional movement through the use of bilateral exercise motion.

8. Improved flexibility and relief of tense muscles.

9. Enhanced social and emotional independence through successful movement.

Arthritis

Arthritis is not necessarily a condition of the aging process. It can occur in the young and old alike. It is characterized by inflammation in and around a joint or joints, usually causing great pain, discomfort, and loss of motion. The degree of arthritic impairment varies from mild inflammation, to swelling and stiffness in joints and connective tissues, to atrophy and debilitating deformities.

Individuals with arthritis can be active and successful participants in water aerobics if certain guidelines are followed. Fatigue is a major curse of arthritis so all exercise periods should start slowly and gradually increase in intensity providing for frequent rest periods. This will help eliminate the stress that can develop from the limited range of motion created by joint inflammation. A minimum water temperature of 84 degrees is suggested. This will help keep the muscles warm and pliable allowing for greater range of motion with the least amount of discomfort.

In general, water aerobics can be of benefit to those with arthritis in the following ways:

1. Increases muscular strength.
2. Increases the range of motion of a joint or joints.
3. Takes the pressure off the joint or joints.
4. Provides an outlet for anxiety created by this form of disability.
5. Provides an exercise medium of warm water that can offer relief to inflamed joints.

Neuromuscular Disorders

Neuromuscular disorders are those which produce weakness or partial paralysis to certain muscles or muscle groups. Impairments of this type are usually caused by infection, heredity, or from certain chronic, progressive diseases such as poliomyelitis, muscular dystrophy, or muscular atrophy.

Exercise for those with neuromuscular diseases need to be of a more moderate nature to decrease the possibility of fatigue. Aerobic workouts may need to be spaced out between flexibility work. For this reason, cardiovascular benefits will be negligible but muscular strength and endurance and flexibility improvement can be achieved. Warmer water of 84 degrees should be maintained to avoid chilling of the muscles and to decrease the chance of muscle cramps.

Water aerobics can benefit the individual with a neuromuscular disorder in the following ways:

1. Provides a medium for organized movement for a longer period of time than attainable on land.
2. Develops muscular strength that will carry over into other daily living activities.
3. Decreases flexion contraction.

4. Increases the joint(s) range of motion.

5. Develops perceptual motor skills and locomotor skills.

6. Strengthens the muscles used for standing and ambulation in the water.

7. Provides an outlet for success and improved self-esteem.

Cerebral Palsy

Cerebral palsy is a dysfunction that can be classified mild to severe. It is usually caused by some degree of damage to the brain when control of the muscles is lost or impaired. The degree of brain damage will determine the extent of muscular damage and adaptation needed for a water aerobics program.

Cerebral palsy is a more debilitating condition than those previously discussed. Sensory input will be low, so movement exploration, including walking, will give the individual a better image and sense of the body in space. Extreme extension, as with any exercise program, should be eliminated. Exercises need to focus on developing strength and endurance. Balance will be seriously affected because of the lack of gravitational pull and buoyancy. The ''buddy system'' should be closely observed since seizures often accompany this condition.

Water aerobics can benefit the individual with cerebral palsy in the following ways:

1. Provides positive relaxation techniques.

2. Stimulates static muscle control and active resistive dynamic motion through the resistive property of water.

3. Provides for the experience of more and freer movement because of the ability to increase the range of motion.

4. Develops motor skills and independent mobility.

5. Utilizes bilateral movement to improve the integration of various movement capabilities.

Multiple Sclerosis

Multiple sclerosis is a disease that affects the central nervous system, not the muscles. It is a chronic, degenerative progressive disease that usually attacks older adolescents and adults. The disease is characterized by numbness, weak limbs, tremors, speech difficulty, fatigue, vision problems, partial paralysis, motor difficulties, spasticity, sensory problems, dizziness and mild emotional disturbances.

Sensory input can be low in the individual, so movement should be done slowly and in a controlled fashion to avoid possible abrasion. Since the onset of fatigue is frequent, exercise periods should be spaced with frequent breaks and rest periods. Overheating should be avoided, so the water temperature should not exceed 84 degrees.

Water aerobics can be a positive experience for the individual with multiple sclerosis in the following ways:

1. Improves muscle tone.
2. Improves ambulation.
3. Improves flexibility, movement capabilities and overall motor control.
4. Improves self-esteem through regular activity.

Cardiac Impairment

Cardiac impairments can be either hereditary or induced through lack of exercise, obesity, stress, and other health related problems. All of these may ultimately result in a heart attack or stroke. Nearly 50% of all the deaths occurring in the United States today are due to heart attacks or strokes.

Before any cardiac patient begins an exercise program, medical approval to begin exercising is required. Workouts should be carefully planned with frequent rest periods and heart rate monitoring. Goals should be set that are attainable and meet the individual's capabilities as well as any medical restrictions. The ''buddy system'' must be strictly enforced so any danger signs such as dizziness, shortness of breath, cyanosis (bluish coloration of the skin caused by a lack of oxygen in the blood), chest pain, and/or irregular heartbeats can be dealt with immediately.

Water aerobics can be a real asset to rehabilitation and the future quality of life for the cardiac impaired individual in the following areas:

1. Relaxing through the choice of music.
2. Increasing cardiovascular endurance gradually.
3. Reducing the anxiety and tension experienced by the post-cardiac patients.
4. Increasing respiration and circulation automatically due to the water pressure.
5. Monitoring and adjusting the activity level according to the patients cardiac condition.

With the increase of heart attacks and strokes in men and women alike, the benefits of a water aerobic exercise program are significant. Any activity that will improve cardiovascular endurance and decrease stress and anxiety, has to ultimately increase and improve the quality of life for the cardiac impaired. Furthermore, starting a water aerobics program now can help prevent cardiac problems in the future.

WARM-UP EXERCISES 5

Warm-up exercises are those exercises that prepare the muscles, ligaments, and tendons for activity. The warm-up used to heat the large muscle groups (legs and arms), reduces the chance of injury. The muscular system is elastic—somewhat like a rubber band. If a rubber band is cold and you pull it, the chance of it breaking is increased. If you warm the rubber band, by gradually stretching it a little farther each time, it will not only become more pliable, the chance of it breaking decreases. Similarly, muscles should be warmed and gradually stretched (static stretch) before exercising.

The warm-up period should begin with a light cardiovascular segment to heat the muscles. In water aerobics, this may include jogging across the pool and back using both a high leg jog and arm pull. Stationary movements involving large muscles such as kicking, hopping, and jumping may also be used. The main purpose of this period is to raise the heart rate slightly and to warm the muscles preparing them for more vigorous exercise.

The warm-up should also include some flexibility exercises. These will stretch the ligaments and tendons decreasing the chance of a sprain or strain to the muscular system. Stretching should include the shoulders, arms, mid-section, back, hips, legs, and feet. All major joints and muscle groups should be included in the flexibility warm-up.

Finally, a muscular strength and endurance segment should be included. Sometimes this portion of the work-out is positioned following the aerobic exercise period. Time availability, in conjunction with adequate warming of the muscles, will determine the placement of this portion of the water aerobic program.

Flexibility Exercises

Shoulder Stretch

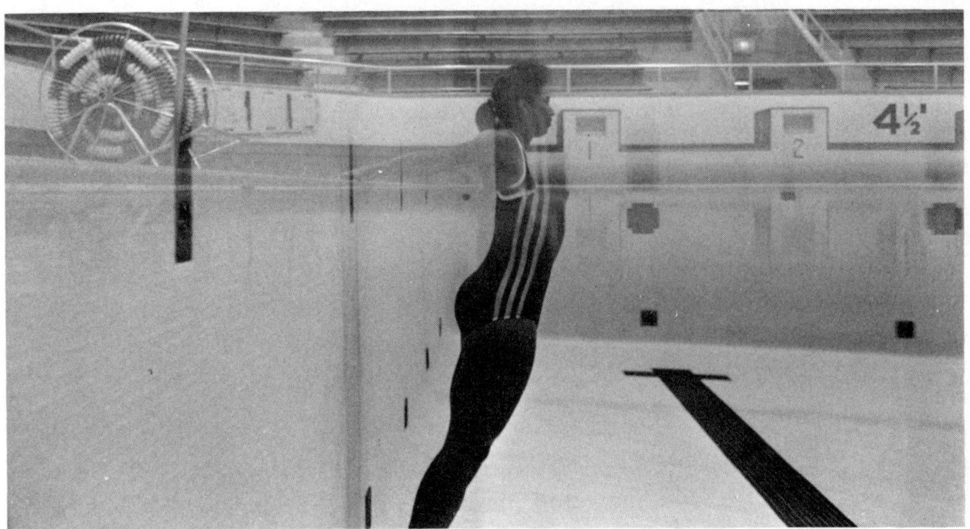

Muscle Groups

Pectorals and Deltoids

Body Position

1. Place hands behind you on the edge of the pool.
2. Hands should be fairly close together to achieve a comfortable stretch.

Execution

1. Walk away from the side of the pool keeping the hands in place.
2. Hold position for 6–10 seconds and repeat.

Key Points

1. Keep the back straight and the feet flat on the bottom of the pool.

Hip Rotation

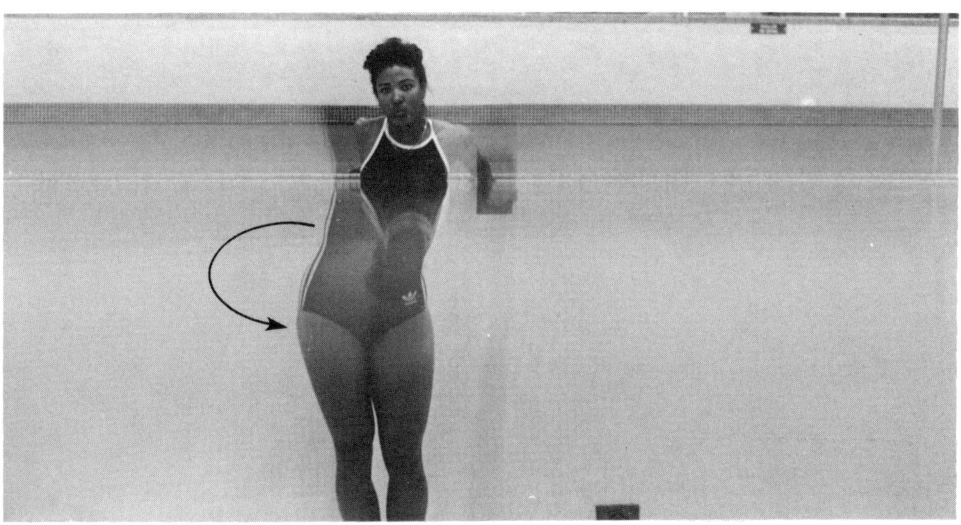

Muscle Groups

Gluteus Maximus and Medius, Lateral and Medial Rotator Groups, and Obliques.

Body Position

1. Turn back to the side of the pool.
2. Place the hands on the side of the pool, behind you and outside the width of the shoulders.
3. Place both feet flat on the bottom of the pool side-by-side and approximately 2 feet from the side of the pool.

Execution

1. Rotate the hips to the right and continue to circle forward, to the left, and behind.
2. Repeat 3–4 times and then repeat an equal number in the other direction.

Key Points

1. Do not over arch the back by thrusting the hips forward.
2. Keep the body aligned over the base of support.
3. The motion should be in the hips, not the upper body.

Leg Press

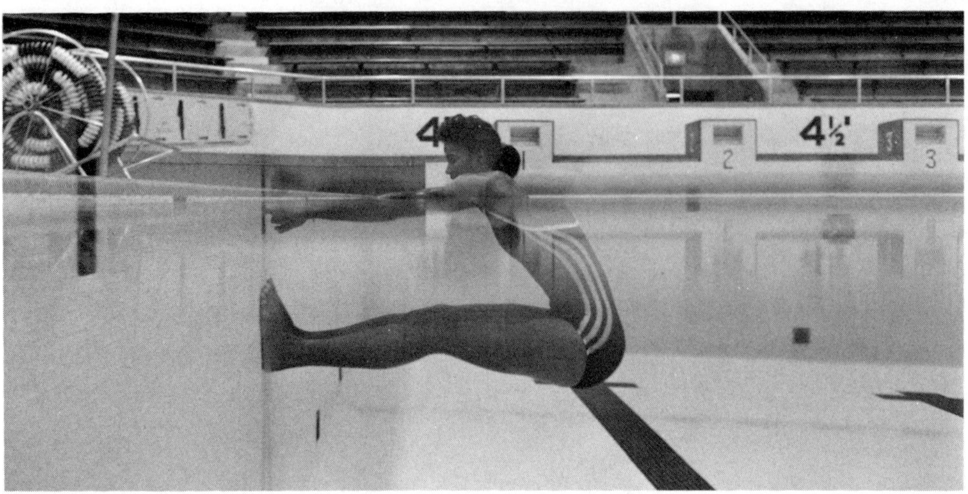

Muscle Groups

Trapezius, Latissimus Dorsi, Hamstrings, Gastrocnemius, Sacrospinalis, Quadriceps, and Gluteus Maximus.

Body Position

1. Face the side of the pool.
2. Place the hands on the side of the pool approximately shoulder width apart.
3. Place the feet together on the side of the pool about a foot below the hands.

Execution

1. Press against the wall of the pool, gradually extending the legs to a comfortable stretch.
2. Hold the position for 6–12 seconds and repeat.

Key Points

1. Do not lock the knees when extending the legs.
2. The stretch should be comfortable for the lower back.

Straight Leg Wall Reach

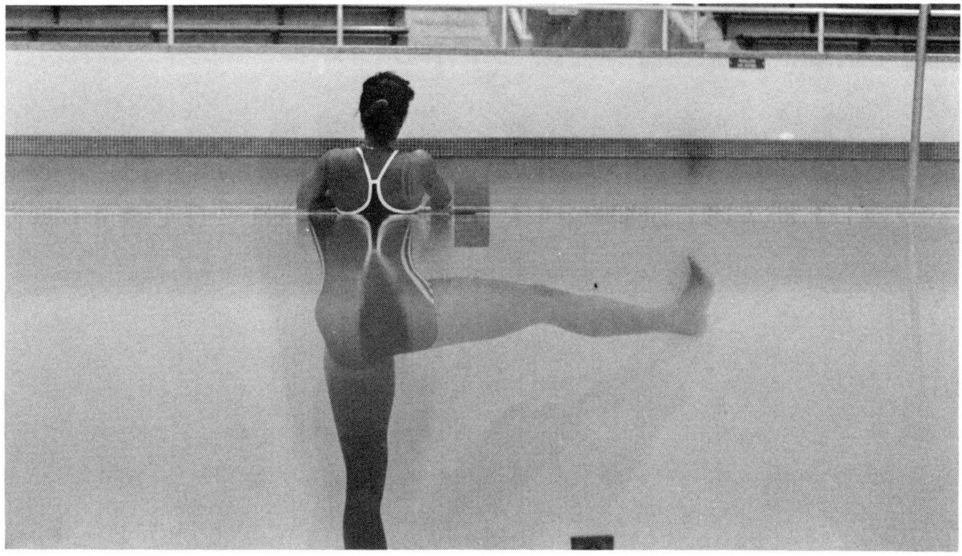

Muscle Groups

Tensor Fasciae Latae, Vastus Lateralis, and Hip Adductors.

Body Position

1. Place the hands shoulder width apart on the top side of the pool.
2. Put the body weight on the left foot with the toe facing the pool and about arms length away from the side.
3. Extend the right leg up to the side and parallel with the side of the pool.
4. Flex the foot on the extended leg so the toes point up.

Execution

1. Pull the extended leg into the wall of the pool.
2. Force the leg back from the thigh and hip, working through the full range of motion.
3. Repeat an equal number of times on each side.

Key Points

1. Keep the extended foot flexed.
2. Keep the body square to the side of the pool throughout the exercise and in good alignment.
3. If the upper leg or hip should cramp, relax the leg and shake it out.

Bent Leg Hip Rotation

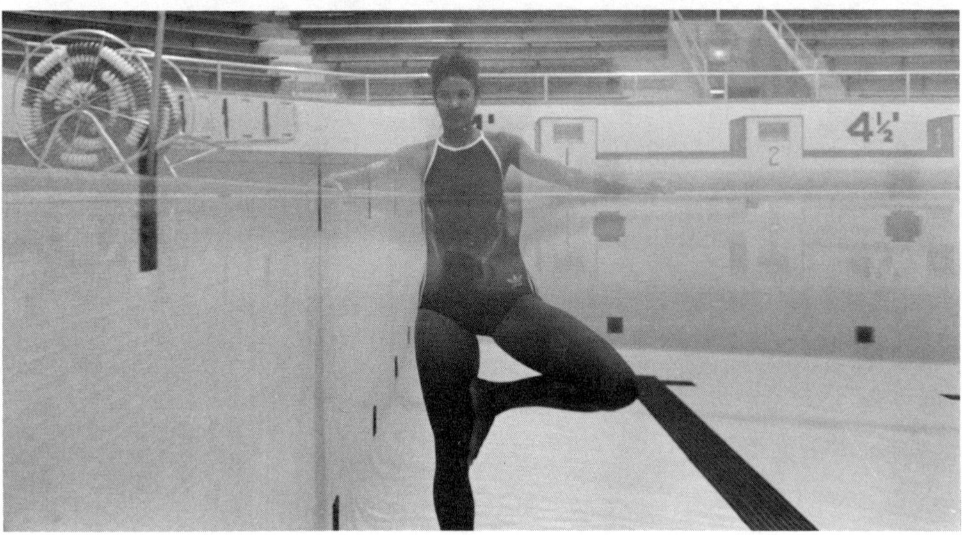

Muscle Groups

Hip Adductors, Tensor Fascia Lata, and Gluteus Medius.

Body Position

1. Place the right hand on the top side of the pool.
2. Face the body perpendicular to the side of the pool.
3. Place the left foot on the inside of the right knee, bending the left knee out to the side.

Execution

1. Pull the bent leg forward from the thigh and hip.
2. Pull the bent leg back to the side position.
3. Repeat an equal number of times on each side.

Key Points

1. Do not pull the bent leg from the knee.
2. Keep the body in good alignment over the support leg.
3. Keep the body still and let the motion occur in the bent leg.

Feet Point and Flex

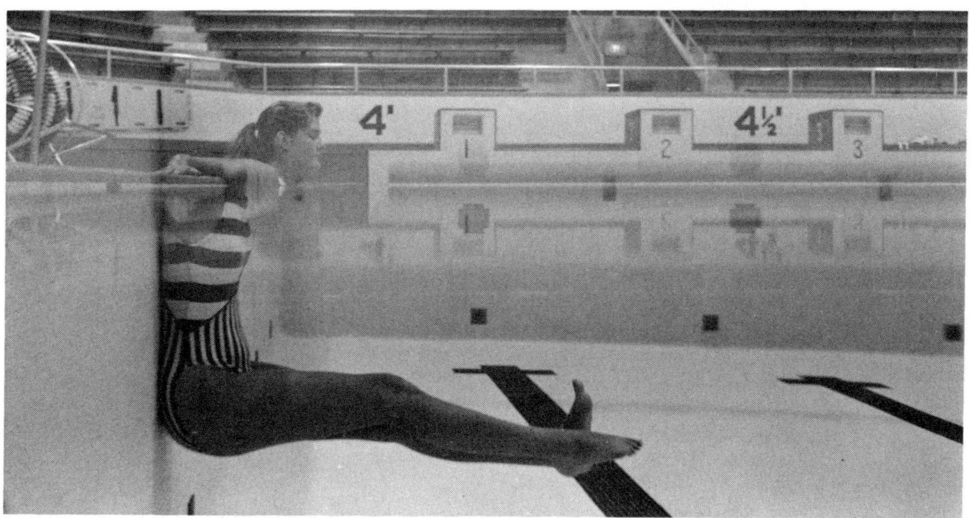

Muscle Groups

Psoas Major, Iliacus, Gastrocnemius, Soleus, Rectus Abdominis, Tibialis Anterior.

Body Position

1. Place the back to the side of the pool.
2. Extend the arms along the top of the pool and drop the body down allowing the buoying effect of the water to support the body.
3. Flatten the back against the side of the pool by tightening the abdominal muscles.
4. Elevate the legs to create a 90 degree angle at the hip.
5. Keep the legs straight in front of the body.

Execution

1. Point the right foot and flex the left foot.
2. Alternate pointing and flexing the feet.

Variations

1. Point or flex both feet at the same time.
2. Rotate the feet at the ankle in both directions.

   1. Keep the back flat against the wall of the pool.
   2. Let the water support the body, not the arms.
   3. Breathe evenly and deeply throughout the exercise.
   4. Do not allow the legs to drop below a 90 degree angle at the hips.

Support Scissors

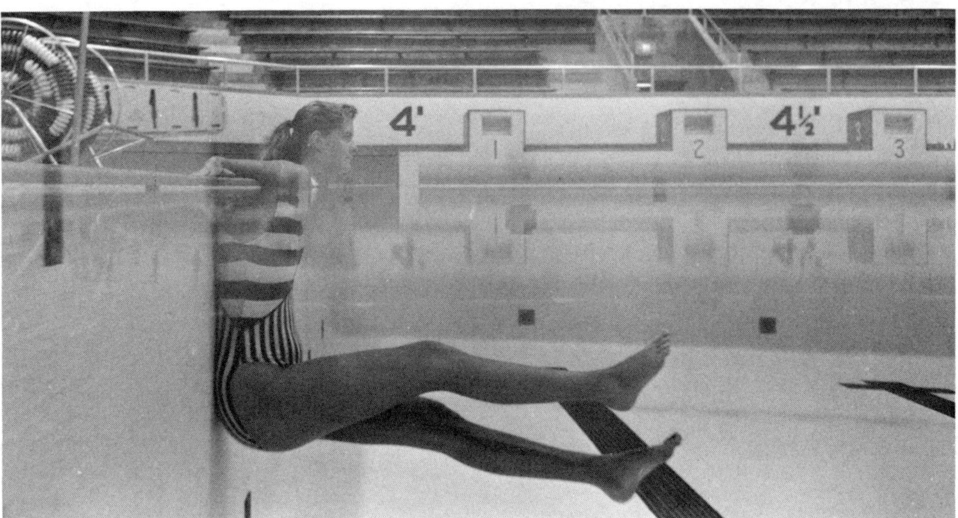

Muscle Groups

Rectus Abdominis, Hip Adductors and Abductors, Fasciae Latae, Vastus Lateralis and Medialis, Psoas Major, and Iliacus.

Body Position

   1. Place the back to the side of the pool.
   2. Extend the arms along the top of the pool and drop the body down allowing the buoying effect of the water to support the body.
   3. Flatten the back against the side of the pool by tightening the abdominal muscles.
   4. Elevate the legs to a 90 degree angle at the hips.
   5. Keep the legs straight in front of the body with the feet relaxed.

Execution

1. Cross the right leg over the top of the left leg.
2. Separate the legs at least shoulder width apart.
3. Cross the left leg over the top of the right leg.
4. Repeat the motion working up to a set of 50–70.

Key Points

1. Keep the back flat against the pool wall.
2. Let the water support the body, not the arms.
3. Breathe evenly and deeply throughout the exercise.
4. Do not allow the legs to drop below a 90 degree angle at the hips.

Support Bent Leg Hip Rotation

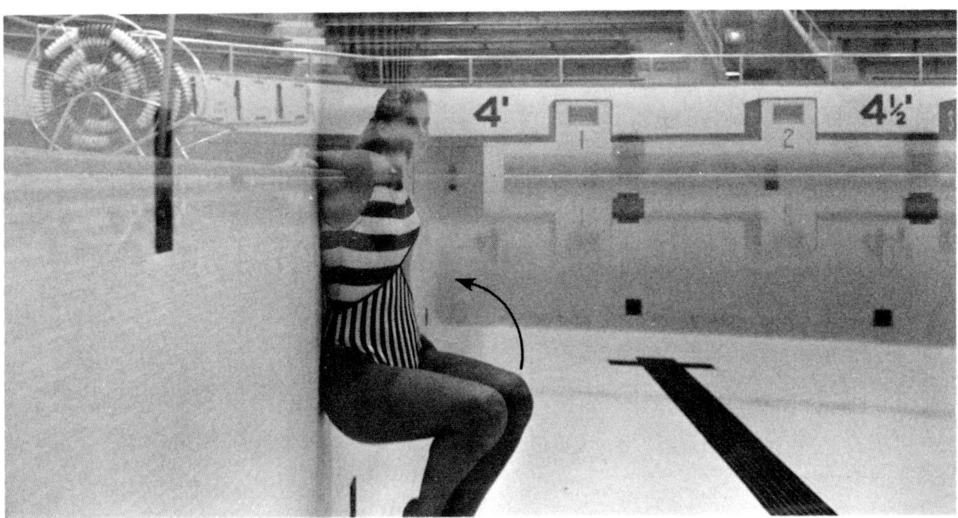

Muscle Groups

Rectus Abdominis, Obliques, Psoas Major, and Iliacus.

Body Position

1. Place the back to the side of the pool.
2. Flatten the back against the side of the pool by tightening the abdominal muscles.
3. Extend the arms along the top of the pool and drop the body down allowing the buoying effect of the water to support the body.
4. Elevate the legs to create a 90 degree angle at the hips.
5. Bend both legs at the knee.

Execution

1. Rotate the legs to the right side at the hip keeping the legs bent.
2. Pull the legs back to the center position and rotate the legs at the hip to the other side.
3. Repeat the motion.

Variations

1. Follow the general body position instructions but keep the legs straight rather than bent. (If you have had any lower back problems do not attempt this variation.)

Key Points

1. Keep the back flat against the pool wall.
2. Let the water support the body not the arms.
3. Breathe evenly and deeply throughout the exercise.
4. Do not allow the legs to drop below a 90 degree angle at the hips.
5. Do not over rotate at the hips placing a strain on the lower back.

Muscular Strength And Endurance

Push Aways

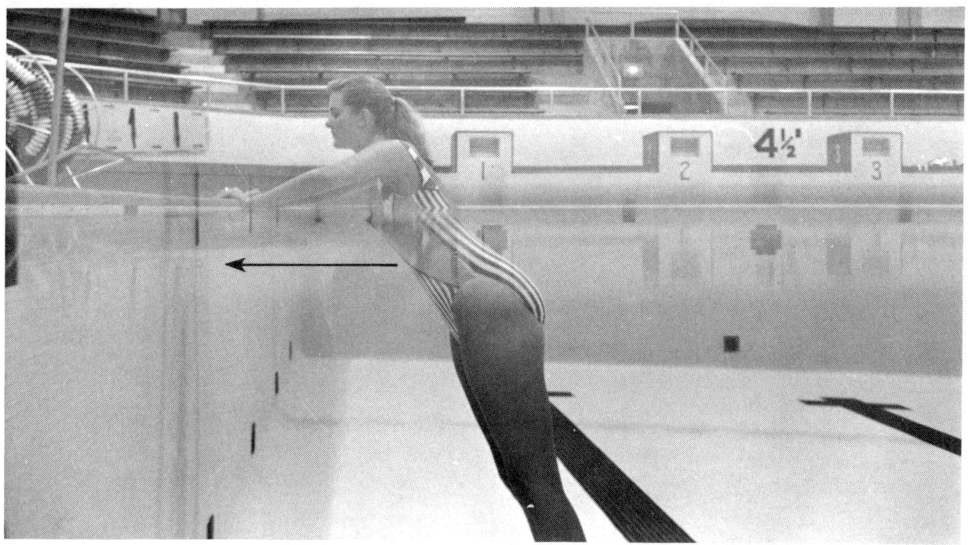

Muscle Groups

Pectorals, Triceps, and Anterior Deltoids.

Body Position

1. Face the side of the pool placing the hands on the top of the pool just outside the width of the shoulders with the arms straight.
2. Place the feet on the bottom of the pool approximately two feet away from the side wall and shoulder width apart.

Execution

1. Let the arms bend to the side as the body leans into the wall.
2. When the body reaches the wall, push it back against the water allowing the arms to straighten.
3. Repeat 10–30 times.

Key Points

1. Keep the body straight with the hips slightly raised.
2. Do not allow the back to arch placing stress on the lower back.
3. Let the heels come off the bottom of the pool on the forward motion.

Front Dips

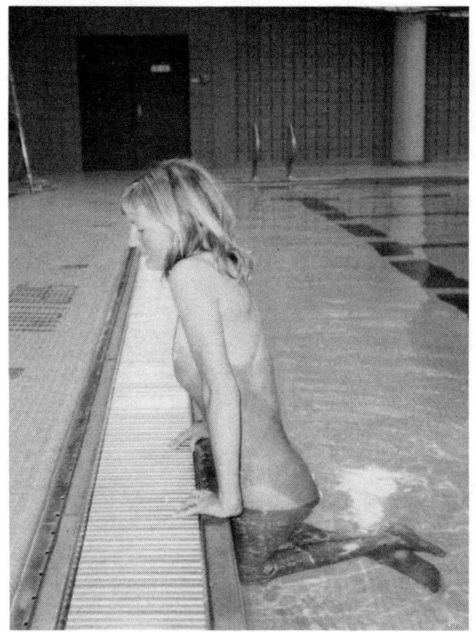

Front Dips—Side View

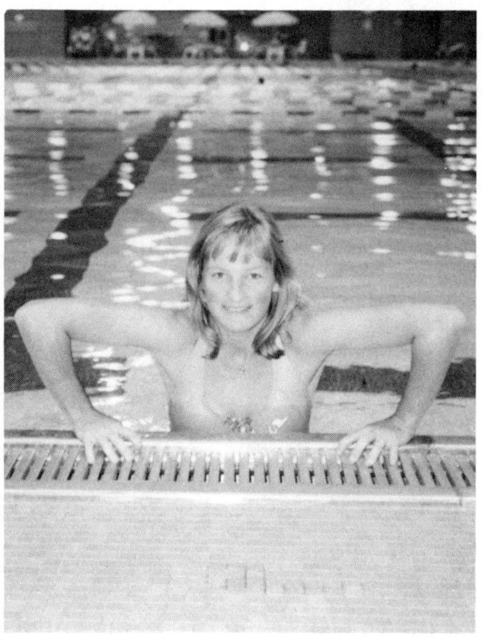

Front Dips—Front View

Muscle Groups

Anterior Deltoids, Trapezius, Triceps, Stabilizors and Rhomboids.

Body Position

1. Face the side of the pool.
2. Place the hands on the top of the pool with the fingers facing forward and the hands on the outside of the shoulders.
3. Keep the arms straight and the shoulders over the hands. Do not allow the body to lean forward.
4. Bend the legs backward at the knees to keep the feet off the bottom of the pool and the body along the side of the pool.

Execution

1. Drop the body from the shoulder to the point where you have a 90 degree angle at the elbow.

2. Push the body back to a straight arm position.

3. Breathe evenly and deeply during the exercise.

Key Points

1. Keep the body straight over the base of support.

2. If the feet float away from the wall when the legs are bent, move to deeper water and keep the legs straight.

3. Do not push off from the bottom of the pool with the feet let the arms do the work.

Back Dips

Muscle Groups

Triceps, and Posterior Deltoids.

Body Position

1. Turn the back to the side of the pool.

2. Place the hands on the top of the pool outside the width of the shoulders with the fingers facing down toward the bottom of the pool.

3. Keep the arms straight.

4. The buttocks and legs should hang down along the side of the pool.

5. You will need to be in chest deep water so the feet do not rest on the bottom of the pool.

Execution

1. Drop the body from the shoulders to the point where there is a 90 degree angle at the elbow.

2. Push the body back up to a straight arm position.

3. Breathe deeply and evenly throughout the exercise.

Key Points

1. Keep the back, buttocks, and legs straight along the side wall.

2. Cross one leg over the other to avoid any kicking motion.

3. Do not push off from the bottom of the pool with the feet let the arms do the work.

Crunch

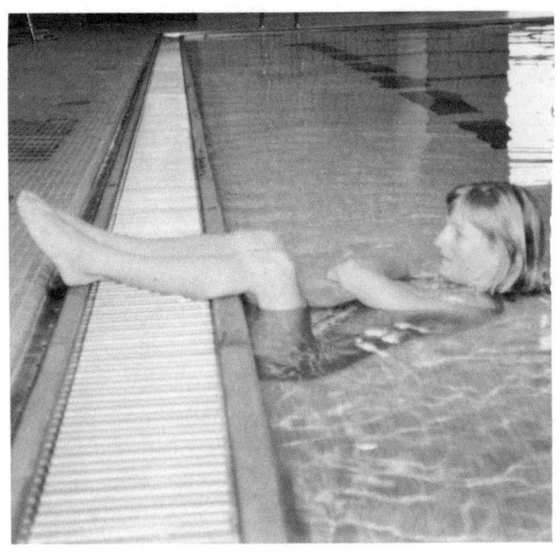

Crunch—Starting Position

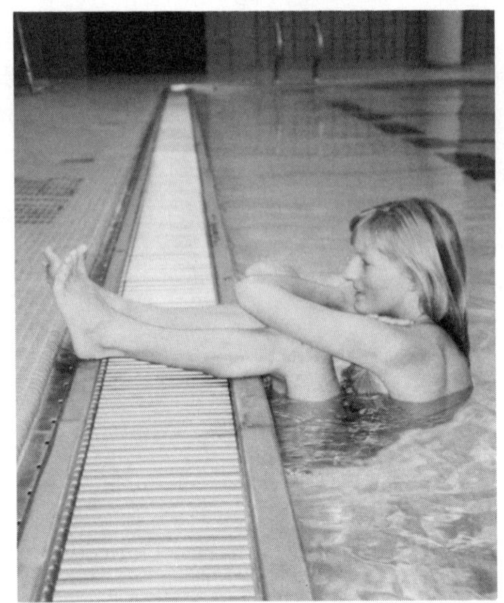

Crunch—Contraction

Muscle Groups

Rectus Abdominis.

Body Position

1. Place both feet and lower legs up on the top of the pool deck. If the legs tend to slide, ask a partner to hold your feet stationary.
2. Press the buttocks flat along the side of the pool.
3. Lay the body back in the water so the nape of the neck is just touching the water.
4. Cross the arms over the chest, holding onto the shoulders with the hands.

Execution

1. Contract the abdominal muscles pulling the body forward.
2. Allow the elbows to pass over the top of the knees.
3. Return to the starting position.

Key Points

1. Keep the buttocks pressed against the wall.
2. Work through the full range of motion.
3. Keep abdominal muscles contracted.

Side Leg Lift

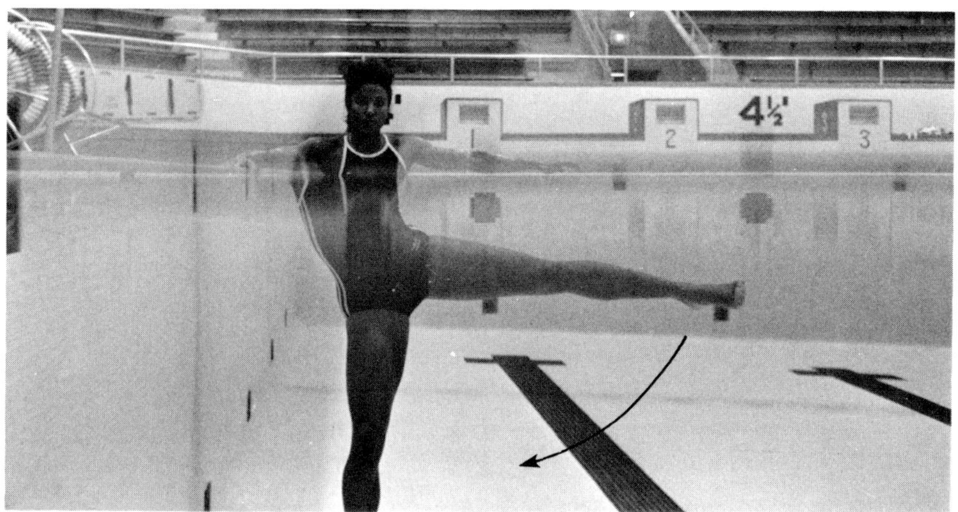

Muscle Groups

Tensor Fasciae Latae, Gluteus Medius and Minimus, Adductor Magnus, Adductor Brevis, Adductor Longus and Pectineus Gracilis.

Body Position

1. Place the right hand on the top of the pool.
2. Face parallel to the side of the pool.
3. Flex the left foot keeping the foot and knee facing forward, not up.
4. Keep the body in alignment over the support leg.

Execution

1. Lift the left leg up to the side keeping the foot flexed forward.
2. Pull the left leg back down by the support leg.
3. Repeat 10–25 times on each leg.

Key Points

1. Work the leg against the water resistance.
2. Keep the body over the support leg.
3. The toe and knee of the working leg must face forward.

AEROBIC EXERCISES

6

The aerobic portion of the exercise program should be at least 20 minutes in length utilizing movements that are continuous and rhythmic in nature. During this time, your heart rate should be raised to the exercise rate and maintained at this level for the entire aerobic exercise period. The intensity level at which you perform the exercises will be determined by your heart rate monitoring during the aerobic segment.

This chapter has been divided into three areas: arm movements, leg movements, and partner work. The arm movements can be interchanged with the leg movements to create a variety of aerobic exercises. Partner work is done for added interest and resistance.

A number of the pictures in this section were taken on land to produce a clearer demonstration of the exercise movement. The line on the wall behind the models reflects the imaginary water line in the pool.

Arm Movements

Figure Eight

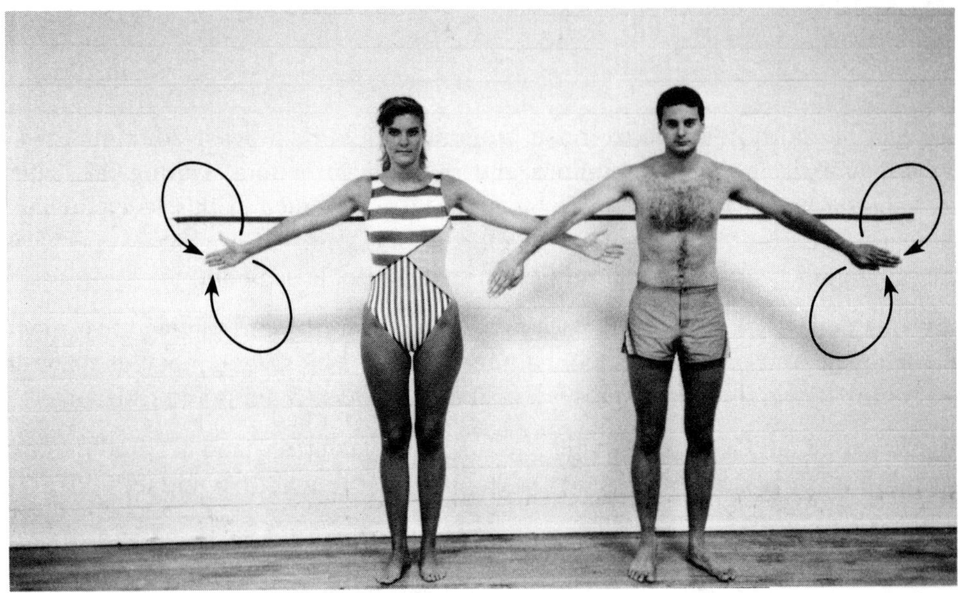

Muscle Groups

Deltoids, Pectorals, and Trapezius.

Body Position

1. Stand in chest deep water.
2. Extend the arms out to the sides at shoulder height.

Execution

1. Move the hands to make a figure eight motion under the water.
2. Use the palm of the hands as a paddle.
3. Make the motion large.

Key Points

1. Keep all the motion under the water.
2. Do not lock the elbows.

One-arm Semi-circles

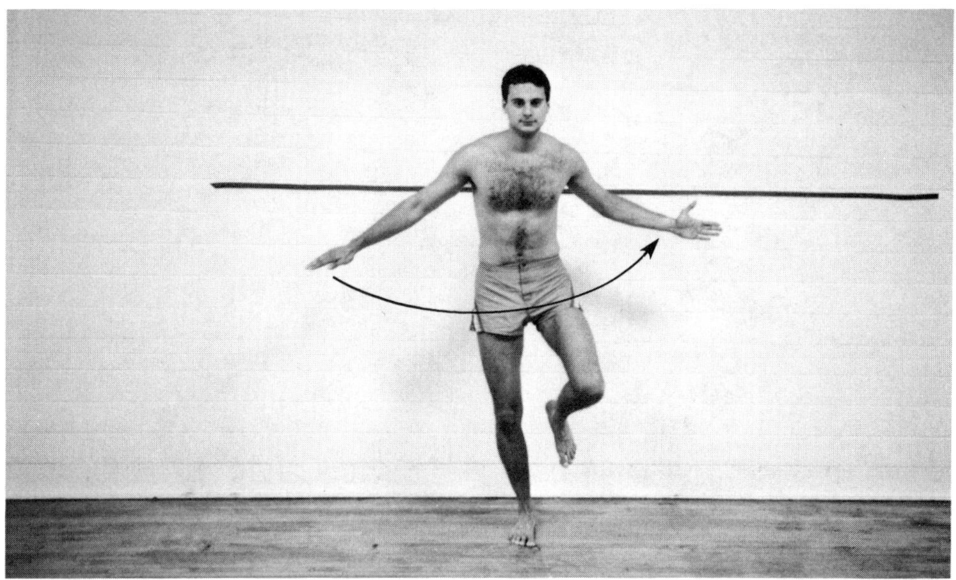

Muscle Groups

Pectorals, Rhomboids, and Latissimus Dorsi.

Body Position

1. Stand in chest deep water.
2. Extend the arms out to the side at shoulders height.

Execution

1. Keep one arm stationary.
2. Pull the other arm over to the stationary arm with the palm of the moving arm toward the stationary arm.
3. Turn the palm of the moving arm over and push the water back to the original position.
4. Work the moving arm through a 180 degree arch.
5. Repeat an equal number of times with each arm.

Key Points

1. Keep the body tall and over the base of support.
2. Use the palm of the moving hand like a paddle.
3. Do not lock the elbows.
4. Keep all the motion under the water.

Front and Back Cross

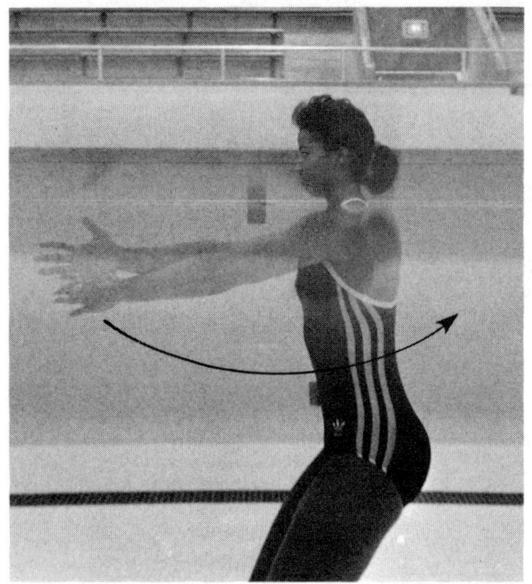

Front Cross

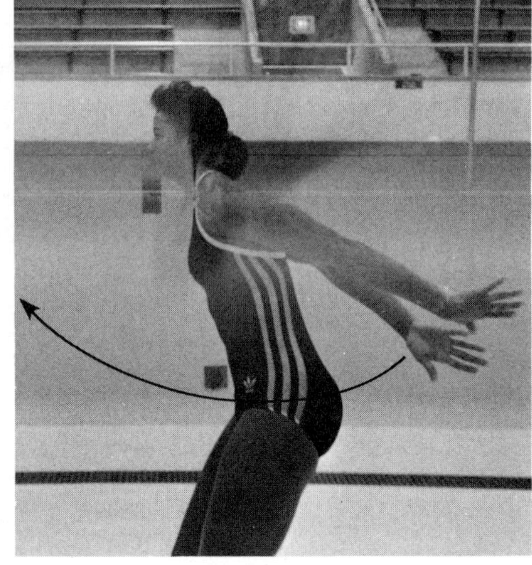

Back Cross

Muscle Groups

Pectorals, Posterior Deltoids, Triceps, Trapezius, and Rhomboids.

Body Position

1. Stand in chest deep water.
2. Extend the arms out to the side at shoulder height.

Execution

1. Face the palms of each hand forward.
2. Pull both arms forcefully forward through the full range of motion crossing the arms in front of the body.
3. Rotate the palm of each hand and push the water all the way back allowing the arms to cross behind the back.
4. Rotate the palms and continue the forward and backward motion.

Key Points

1. Keep all the motion under water.
2. Work the arms through the full range of motion.
3. Do not lock the elbows.

Elephant Trunk

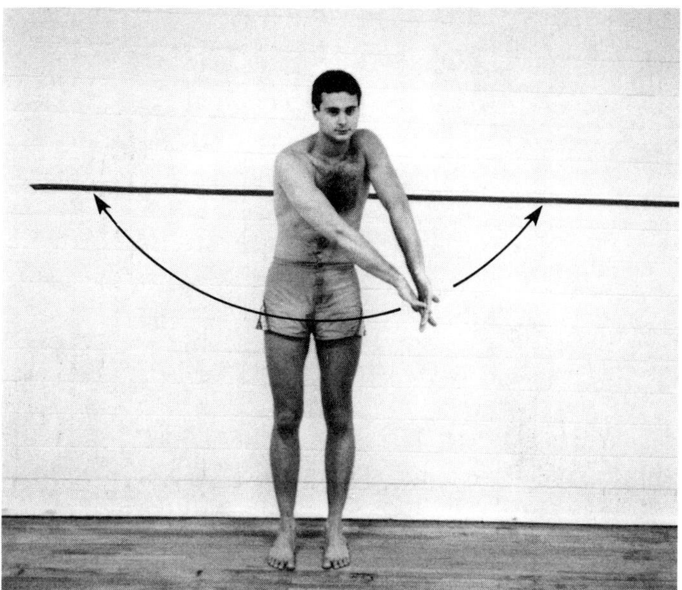

Muscle Groups

Triceps, Deltoids, and Latissimus Dorsi.

Body Position

1. Stand in chest deep water.
2. Join the hands with the fingers interlocked and the hands back to back, palms facing out to the sides.

Execution

1. Extend the arms down in front of the body with the hands interlocked at the fingers as explained above.
2. Push the right palm up toward the right side carrying the arms close to the water surface.
3. Push the left palm down and up to the left side carrying the arms close to the water surface.
4. Repeat swinging motion equally on both sides.

Key Points

1. Keep the body tall and do not bend forward at the waist.
2. Work the arms like a pendulum.
3. Keep the arms straight but do not lock the elbows.

Push and Pull Arm Circles

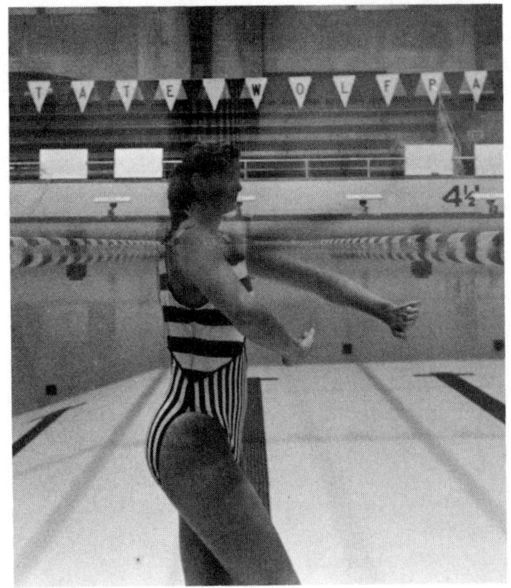

Palm Push

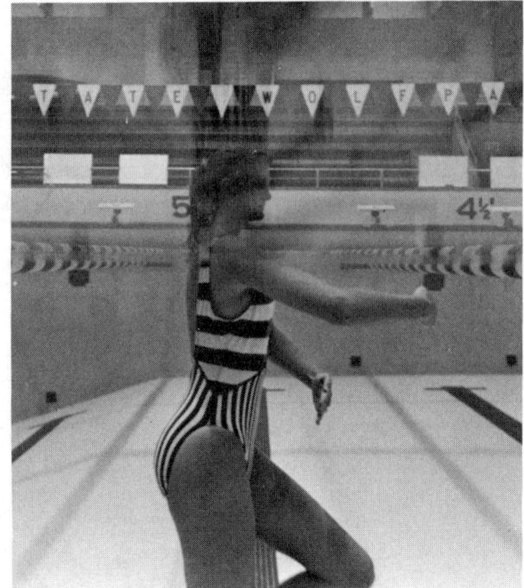

Palm Pull

Muscle Groups

Carpi (Wrist) Flexors and Extensors,. Biceps, Triceps, and Brachials.

Body Position

1. Stand in chest deep water.
2. Keep the arms out in front of the body at shoulder height to chest height.

Execution

1. Face the palm of each hand away from the body.
2. Push the water away with the right palm by extending the arm forward.
3. Pull the back of the opposite hand toward the body.
4. Repeat the motion allowing the hands to circle around each other as you push and pull.
5. Face the palm of each hand toward the body and repeat the motion.

Key Points

1. Work arms through the full range of motion and full arm extension.
2. Keep all motion under the water.

Side Reach and Pull

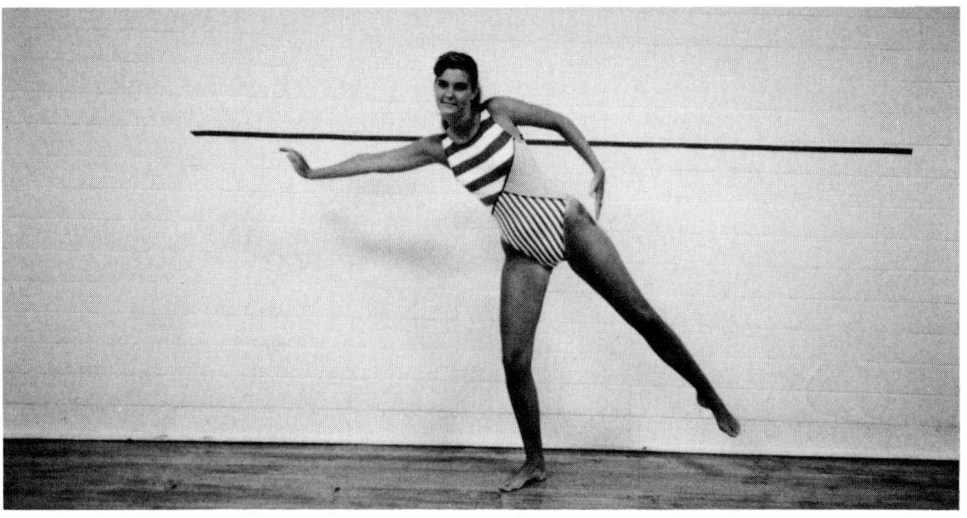

Muscle Groups

Obliques, Latissimus Dorsi, Trapezius, Deltoids, and Carpi (Wrist) Flexors and Extensors.

Body Position

1. Stand in chest deep water.
2. Extend one arm out to the side at shoulder height.
3. Keep the opposite arm bent at the side of the body.

Execution

1. Push the water away with the palm of the bent arm hand at shoulder height, reaching as far as possible to the side.
2. Pull the water toward the body with the extended arm.
3. Repeat the reaching and pulling motion from side to side.

Key Points

1. Push the reaching arm out as far as possible.
2. Water should rush by the hip on the pulling motion.
3. Keep all motion under the water.

Front Arm Push and Pull

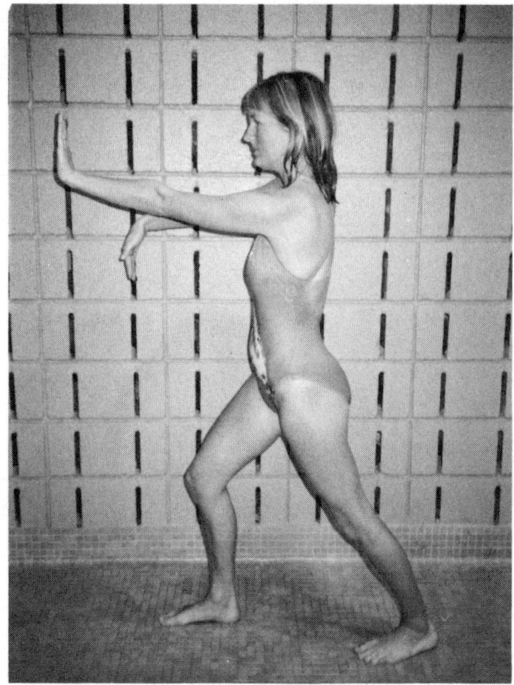

Muscle Groups

Trapezius, Pectorals, and Carpi (Wrist) Flexors and Extensors.

Body Position

1. Stand in chest deep water.
2. Extend one arm out in front of the body at shoulder height with the palm facing forward.

Execution

1. Point fingers of extended arm down with the palm toward the body and pull the water to the chest.
2. Push the opposite arm out in front with the palm facing out extending the arm at shoulder height.
3. Repeat the pulling and pushing motion.

Key Points

1. Make sure to change the hand position at the wrist.
2. Extend the arm fully on the pushing motion.
3. Keep the body tall and do not bend at the waist.

Pumping Up

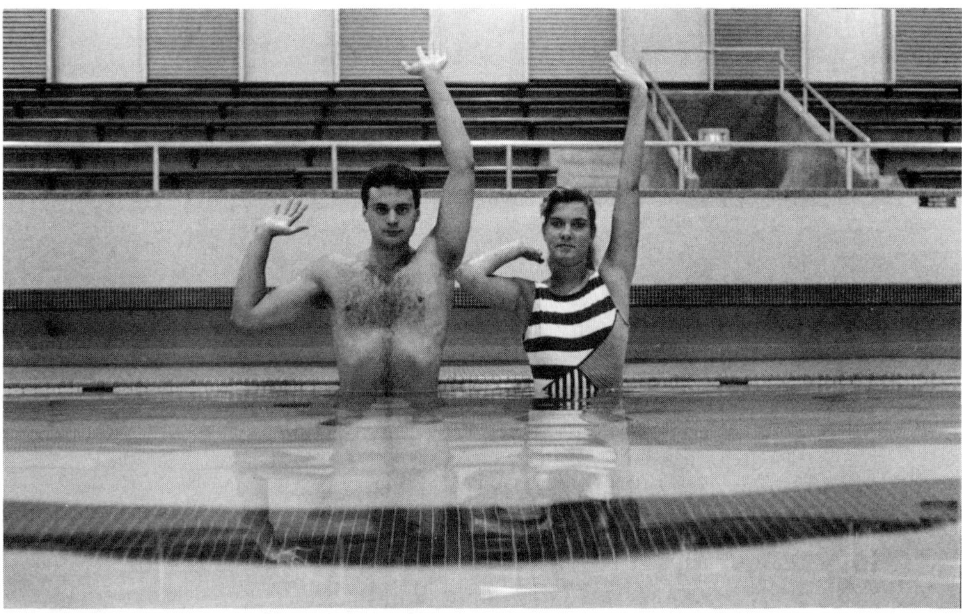

Muscle Groups

Anterior and Medial Deltoids, Trapezius, Triceps, and Serratus Anterior.

Body Position

1. Stand in chest deep water.
2. Extend the arm straight up over the shoulder but do not lock the elbow.
3. Bend the opposite arm at the elbow with the palm of the hand facing up.

Execution

1. Extend the bent arm by pushing the palm of the hand upward.
2. Drop the opposite arm down to the shoulder by bending it at the elbow and keeping the palm up.
3. Repeat the motion alternating the arms.

Key Points

1. Keep the body standing tall.
2. Reach as high as possible.
3. Do not lock the elbows when the arm is extended.

Arm Sway

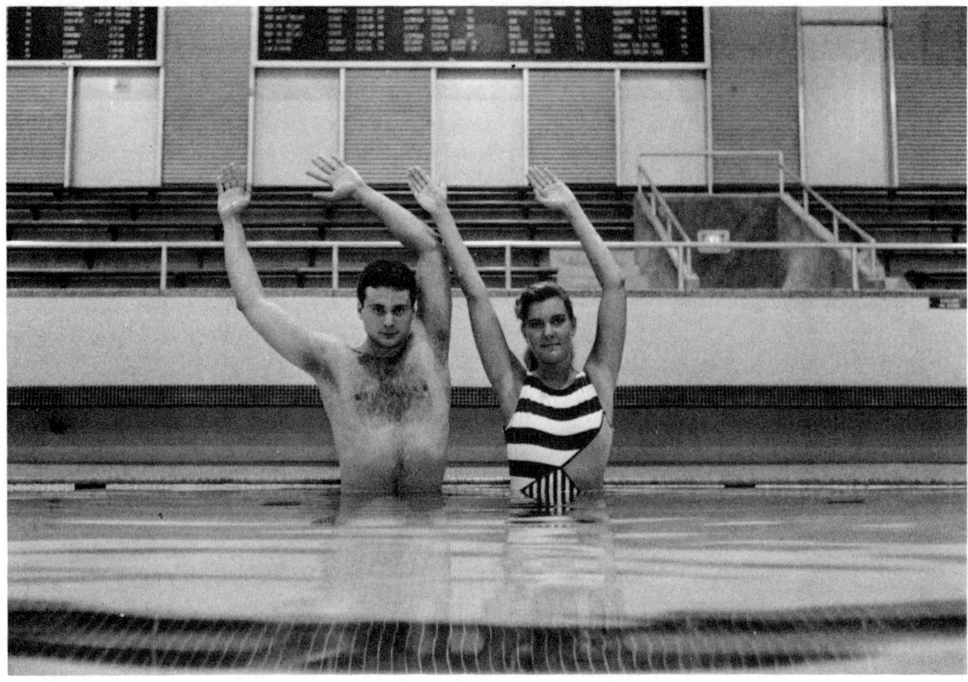

Muscle Groups

Latissimus Dorsi and Medial Deltoids.

Body Position

1. Stand in chest deep water.
2. Extend both arms up over the head and shoulders.

Execution

1. Sway both arms over the head and to the right.
2. Repeat the motion to the left.

Key Points

1. Allow the arms to sway from the shoulders, not from the elbow.
2. Keep the arms high and the body tall.

Leg Movements

Jog

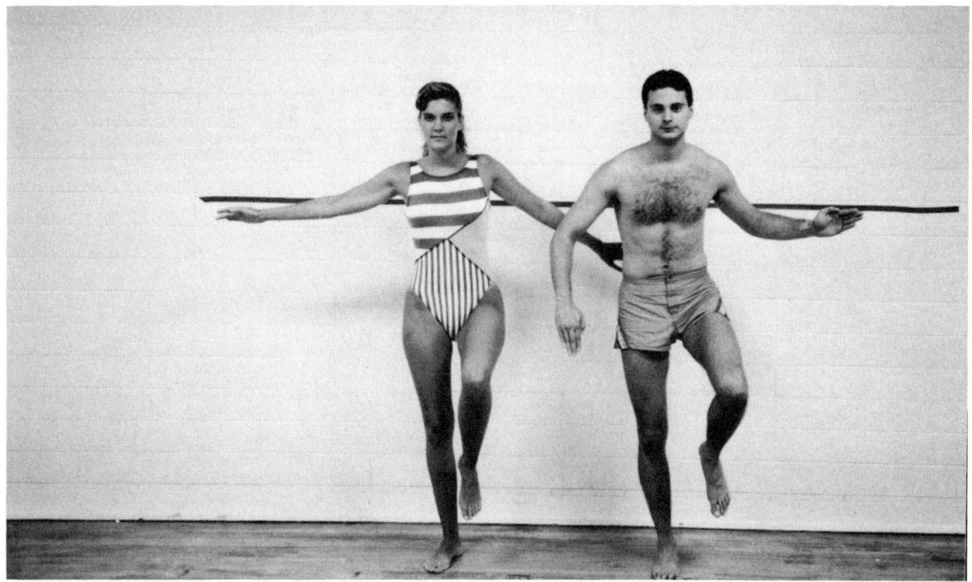

Muscle Groups

Total body workout.

Body Position

1. Stand in chest deep water.
2. Elevate one leg to form a 90 degree angle at the hip and knee.

Execution

1. Briskly alternate the leg lift, pushing off the bottom of the pool with the support foot.

Key Points

1. Keep the body tall and in good alignment.
2. Push the water up toward the surface with the thigh.
3. Do not bend in the middle.
4. Push off the bottom of the pool with a flat foot.
5. Do not lock the knee of the support leg.

Lower Leg Circles

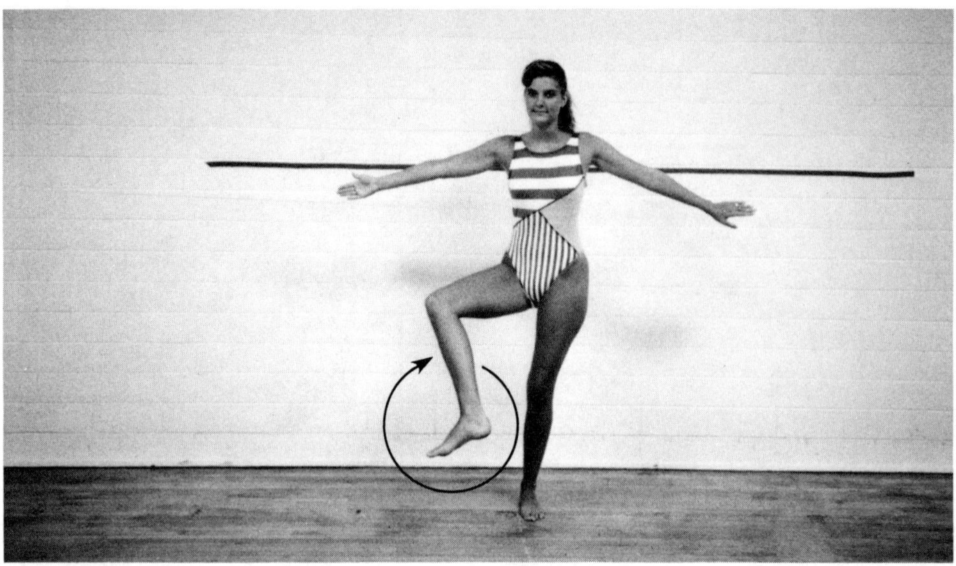

Muscle Groups

Gracilis, Iliopsoas, and Hip Flexors.

Body Position

1. Stand in chest deep water.
2. Support the weight on one leg.
3. Rotate the thigh of the other leg to the outside and bend the leg at the knee.

Execution

1. Keep the foot of the bent knee flexed.
2. Make a circle with the lower leg.
3. Repeat motion several times and change legs.

Key Points

1. Do not over rotate the lower leg.
2. If discomfort is felt in the knee, discontinue the exercise.
3. Push the water around with the arch of the flexed foot.
4. Do not lock the knee of the support leg.

Wide Side Leg Hop

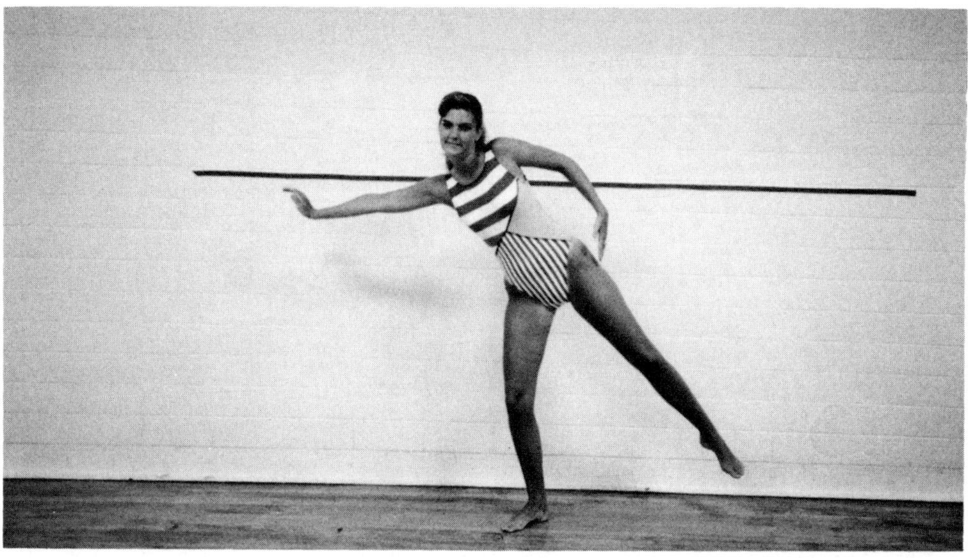

Muscle Groups

Adductor Magnus and Longus, Gluteus Maximus, Tensor Fasciae Latae, Gastrocnemius, and Soleus.

Body Position

1. Stand in chest deep water.
2. Separate the feet wide to both sides.

Execution

1. Push off the bottom of the pool with the right foot.
2. With the legs wide, land on the left foot.
3. Repeat the motion off the left foot.

Key Points

1. Keep the feet wide and well outside the width of the shoulders.
2. Keep the motion side-to-side.
3. Push off the bottom with a flat foot.

Frog Legs

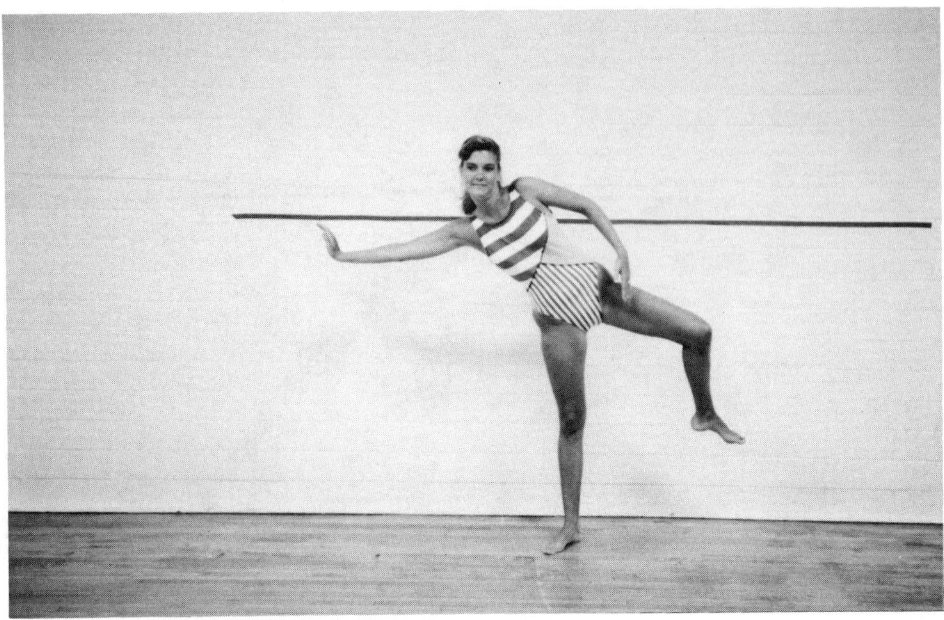

Muscle Groups

Hip Abduction, Tensor Fasciae Latae, and Gluteus Medius and Minimus.

Body Position

1. Stand in chest deep water.
2. Support the body weight on one leg.
3. Bend the opposite leg at the knee, rotating the thigh to the side.

Execution

1. Maintain the thigh turn-out throughout the exercise.
2. Push off the bottom of the pool with the support foot.
3. Transfer the weight to the other leg keeping the turn-out at the thigh.
4. Repeat the sequence alternating legs.

Key Points

1. Keep a wide turn-out at the thigh.
2. Keep the toes facing to the side to assist in the turn-out.

Heel Slap

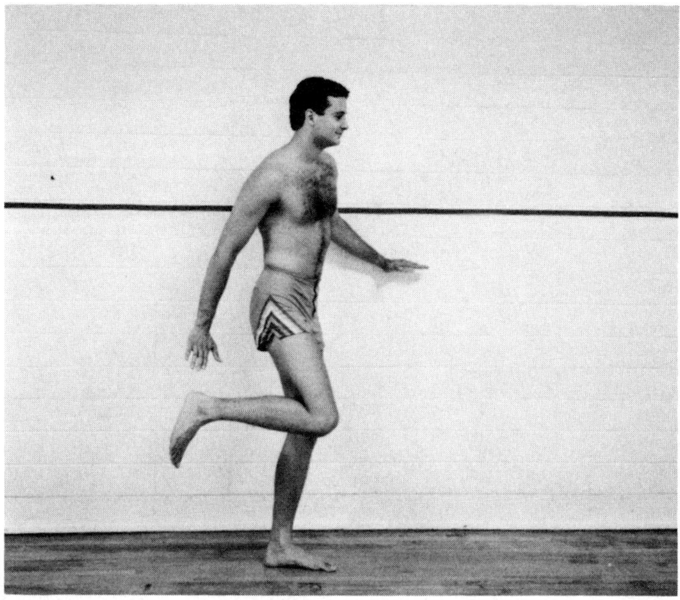

Muscle Groups

Gastrocnemius, Hamstrings, Soleus, and Tibialis Anterior.

Body Position

1. Stand in chest deep water.
2. Support the body weight on the left leg.
3. Bend the right leg up behind the body at the knee.
4. Flex the foot of the bent knee.

Execution

1. Force the right hand down toward the heel of the right foot.
2. Transfer the weight to the right leg as you bring the heel of the left foot up in back and the left hand down toward the heel of the left foot.
3. Repeat, alternating the legs and the up-and-down motion with the arms.

Key Points

1. Work the hands up and down behind the body keeping the elbows high and the palms down.
2. Keep the support foot flat on the bottom of the pool.
3. Lift the bent leg from the heel, not the knee.
4. Keep the body in good alignment over the support leg.
5. Do not lock the knee of the support leg.

Low Kicks

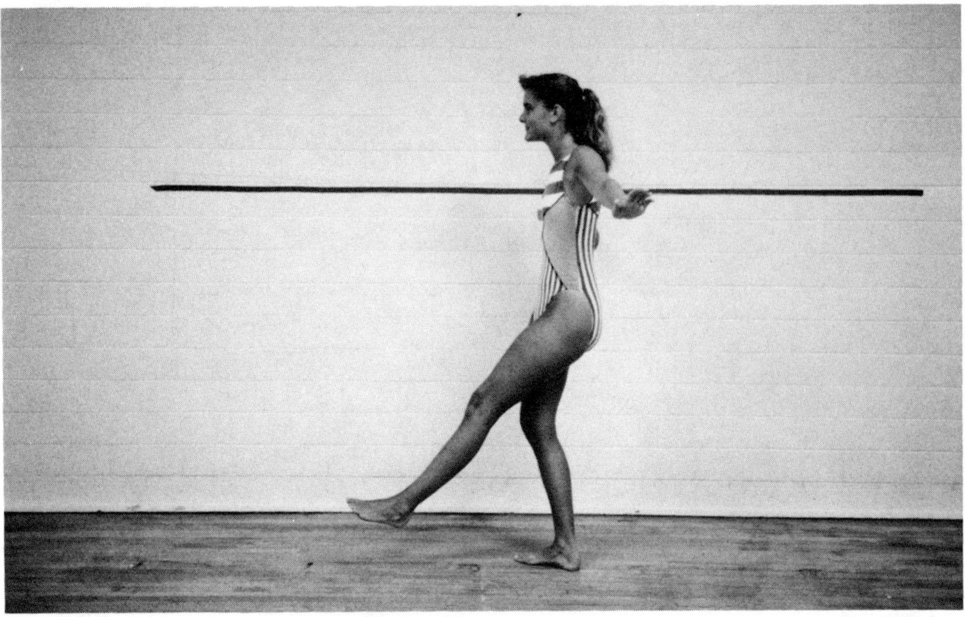

Muscle Groups

Hip Extensors, Tibialis Anterior, Iliopsoas, Gastrocnemius, and Soleus.

Body Position

1. Stand in chest deep water.
2. Support the body weight on the right leg.
3. Extend the left leg out in front of the body from the hip.

Execution

1. In one movement, transfer the body weight to the left leg and from the hip kick the right leg out in front of the body.
2. Kick the leg about 12–18 inches off the bottom of the pool.
3. Repeat alternating the kicking leg.

Key Points

1. Keep the foot of the kicking leg relaxed.
2. Keep the body tall and in good alignment.
3. Make sure to kick the leg from the hip, not the knee.
4. Do not lock the knee of the support leg.

High Kicks

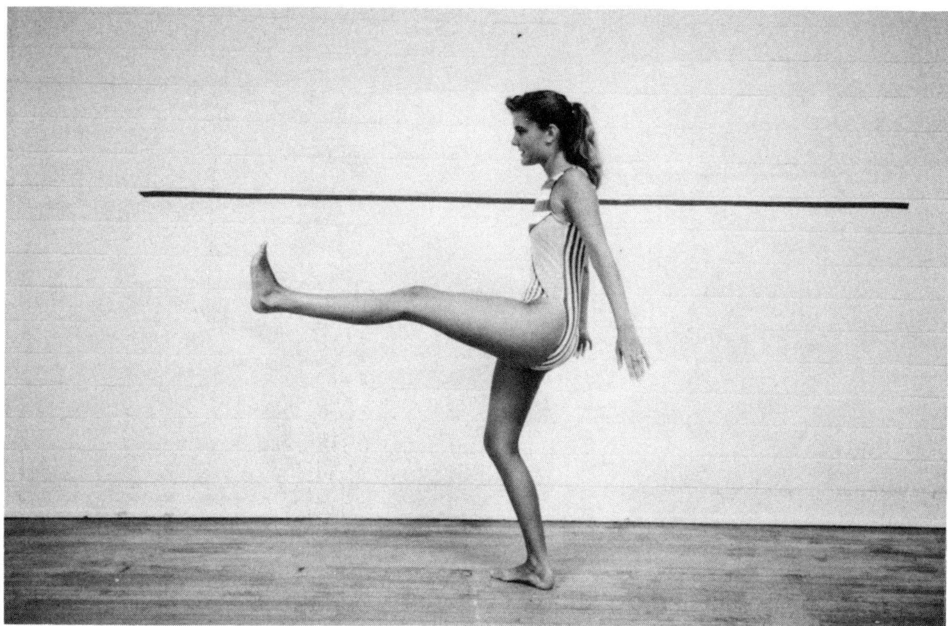

Muscle Groups

Hip Flexors, Gluteus Maximus and Medius, Psoas Major, Iliacus, and Gastrocnemius.

Body Position

1. Stand in chest deep water.
2. Support the weight on the right leg.

Execution

1. From the hip, kick the left leg high out in front of the body.
2. Pull the left leg down to become the support leg as you kick the right leg high in front of the body.
3. Repeat alternating the legs.

Key Points

1. Do not lock the knee of the kicking or supporting leg.
2. Keep the body tall and in good alignment.
3. Kick the leg from the hip, not the knee.

Bend and Kick

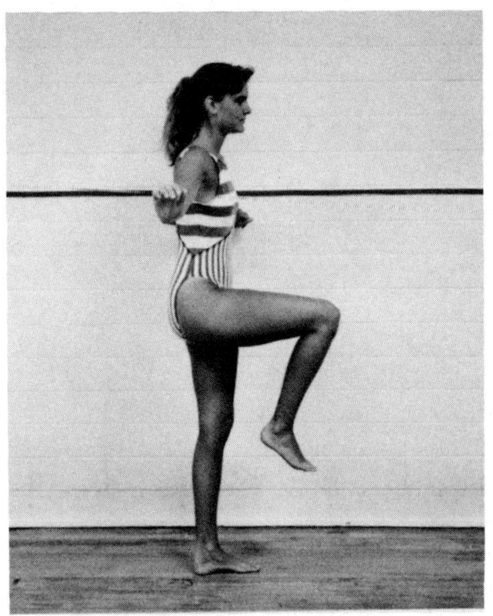

Bend and Kick—Knee Lift

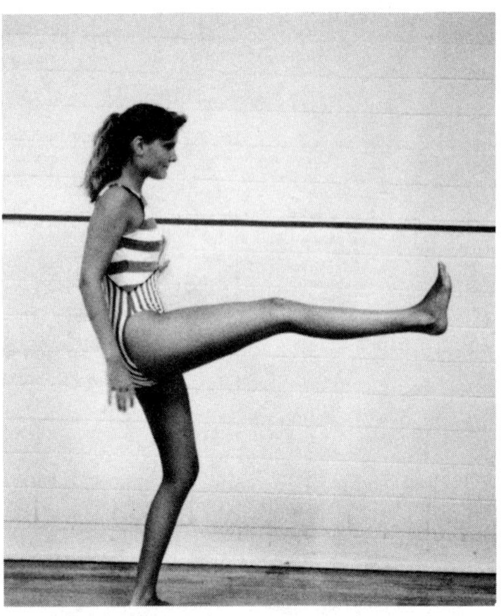

Bend and Kick—High Kick

Muscle Groups

See Jog and High Kick.

Body Position

1. Stand in chest deep water.
2. Bend the right leg at the knee in front of the body.
3. Support the body weight on the left leg.

Execution

1. Hop on the support leg.
2. Lower the bent leg and then, from the hip, kick it out in front of the body.
3. Hop on the support leg.
4. Change legs and continue the exercise, alternating legs and the bend-hop-kick-hop motion.

Key Points

1. Do not lock the knee of the support leg.
2. Keep the body tall and in good alignment.

One Leg Hop-and-Hold

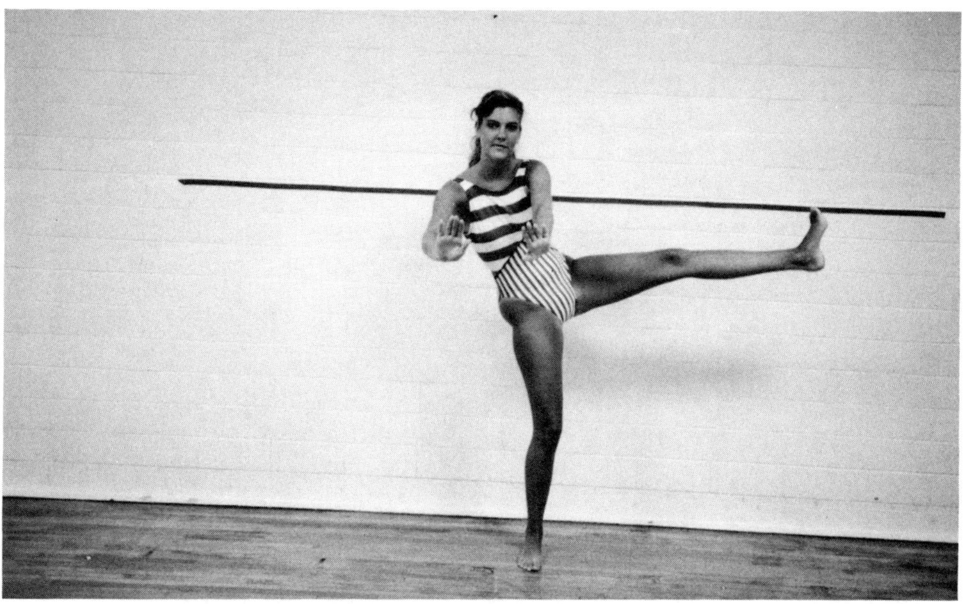

Muscle Groups

Gluteus Maximus, Tensor Fasciae Latae, Hip Abduction, Gastrocnemius, and Quadriceps.

Body Position

1. Stand in chest deep water.
2. Support the body weight on the right leg.
3. Extend the left leg up to the side with the foot flexed toward the ceiling or sky.

Execution

1. Hop on the right leg.
2. Hold the left leg up to the side.
3. Repeat the motion several times, then change legs.

Key Points

1. Keep the body tall and in good alignment.
2. Do not lock the knees.
3. Keep the foot flexed on the extended leg.

Bent Leg Hop

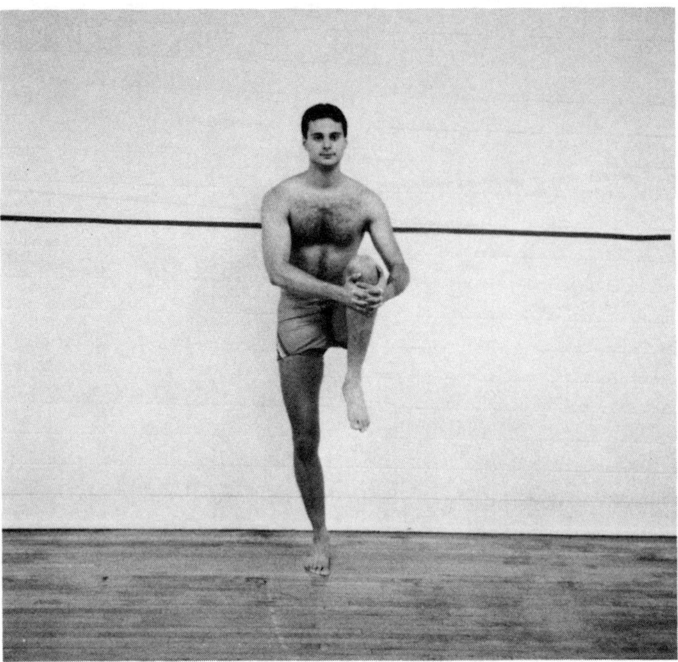

Muscle Groups

Quadriceps, Gastrocnemius, and Soleus.

Body Position

1. Stand in chest deep water.
2. Support the body weight on the right leg.
3. Bend the left leg up and hug it close to the chest.

Execution

1. Hop on the right leg while holding the left leg bent and close to the chest.
2. Repeat several times and change legs.

Key Points

1. Do not lock the knee of the support leg.
2. Hop off of a flat foot.
3. Keep the body tall and in good alignment.
4. If you have hand knee problems or feel discomfort in the bent leg knee, hold the leg behind the thigh rather than in front of the knee.

Cross Country Ski

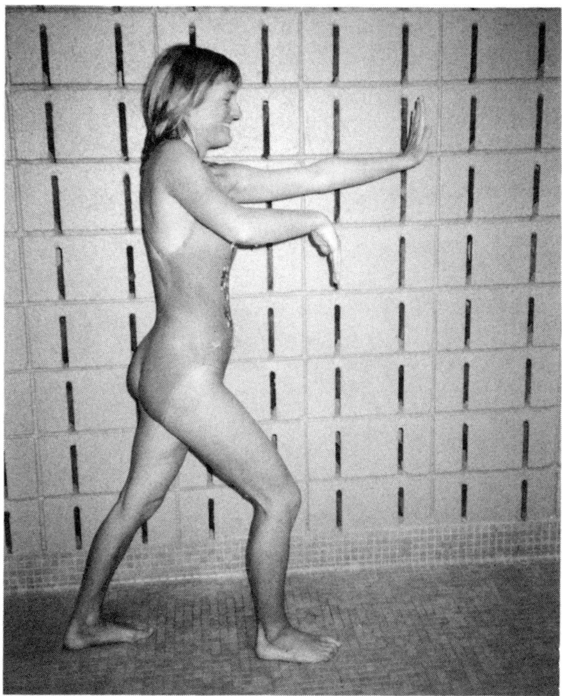

Muscle Groups

Hip Flexors, Hip Extensors, and Gluteus Maximus.

Body Position

1. Stand in chest deep water.
2. Extend the right leg out in front of the body with the foot flat on the bottom of the pool.
3. Reach behind with the left leg placing the foot on the bottom of the pool.

Execution

1. Quickly alternate the position of the feet.
2. Repeat the sequence alternating the feet position.
3. Keep the legs wide to achieve a comfortable stretch.

Key Points

1. Keep the body tall and in good alignment.
2. Do not lock the knees.
3. Keep the feet as flat as possible on the bottom of the pool.

Jumping Jacks

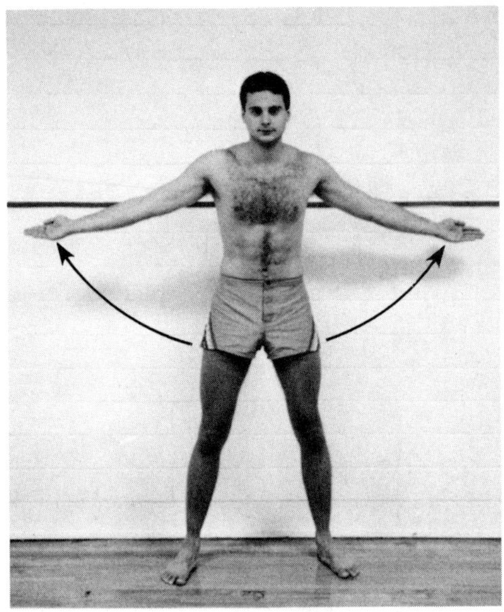

Jumping Jacks—Open

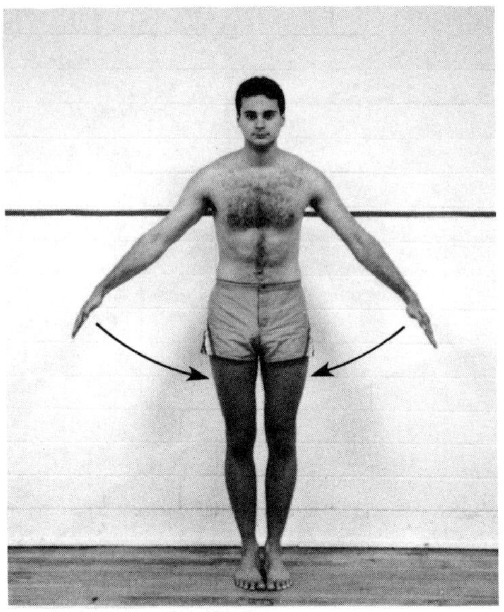

Jumping Jacks—Close

Muscle Groups

Hip Adductors and Abductors, and Shoulder Adductors and Abductors.

Body Position

1. Stand in chest deep water.
2. Separate the feet to the side just outside the width of the shoulders.
3. Extend the arms out to the side of the body close to the water surface with the palms facing up.

Execution

1. Turn the palms of the hands down and pull the arms to the sides of the body.
2. Whip the legs together in conjunction with the arm motion.
3. Turn the palms of the hands up and push the arms up close to the water surface.
4. Whip the legs out to the sides of the body in conjunction with the arm motion.
5. Repeat the open and close motion.

Key Points

1. Do not lock the knees or elbows.
2. Do not break the surface of the water with the hands.
3. Keep the body tall and in good alignment.

Scissors

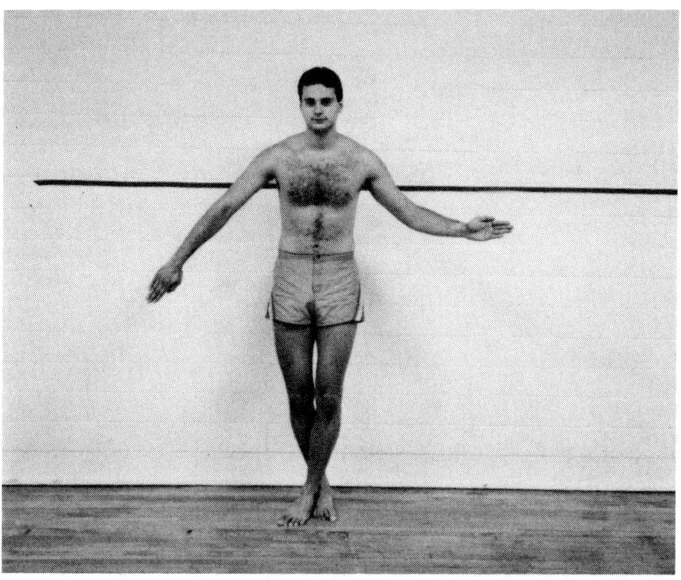

Muscle Groups

Hip Adductors and Abductors, Gluteus Maximus, Tensor Fasciae Latae, Gastrocnemius, and Soleus.

Body Position

1. Stand in chest deep water.
2. Cross the left leg in front of the right leg keeping both feet flat on the bottom of the pool.

Execution

1. Quickly push off the bottom of the pool with both feet.
2. Separate the feet about shoulder width apart. forcefully.
3. Whip the legs back, crossing the right leg in front of the left.
4. Place both feet back on the bottom of the pool with the legs crossed.
5. Repeat the sequence.

Key Points

1. Keep the body tall and in good alignment.
2. Do not lock the knees.
3. Forcefully separate the legs and whip them back.

The Twist

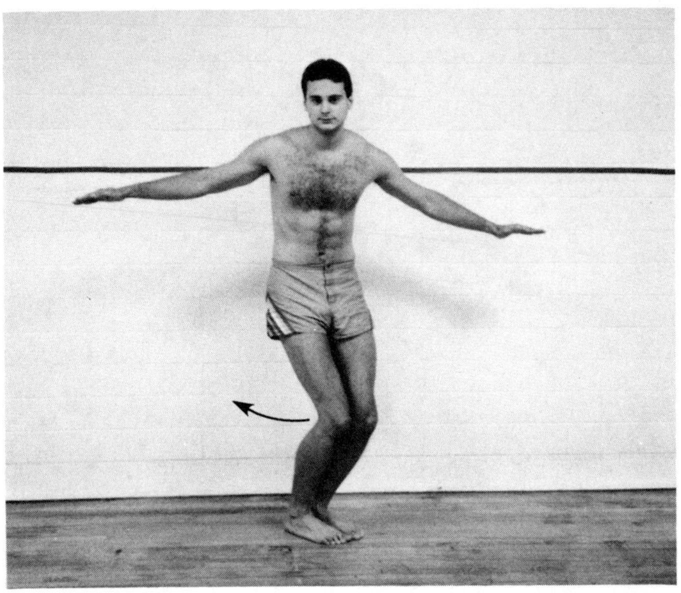

Muscle Groups

Internal and External Obliques.

Body Position

1.   Stand in chest deep water.
2.   Place feet together on the bottom of the pool.
3.   Bend the knees slightly.

Execution

1.   Rotate the hips and waist to the left allowing the legs and feet to follow the motion.
2.   Rotate the hips and waist to the right allowing the legs and feet to follow the motion.
3.   Repeat the motion, alternating from side-to-side.

Key Points

1.   Keep the body tall and in good alignment.
2.   Keep the upper body still, allowing the motion to occur from the waist down.
3.   Keep the feet flat on the bottom of the pool.

Partner Movements

Swing Your Partner

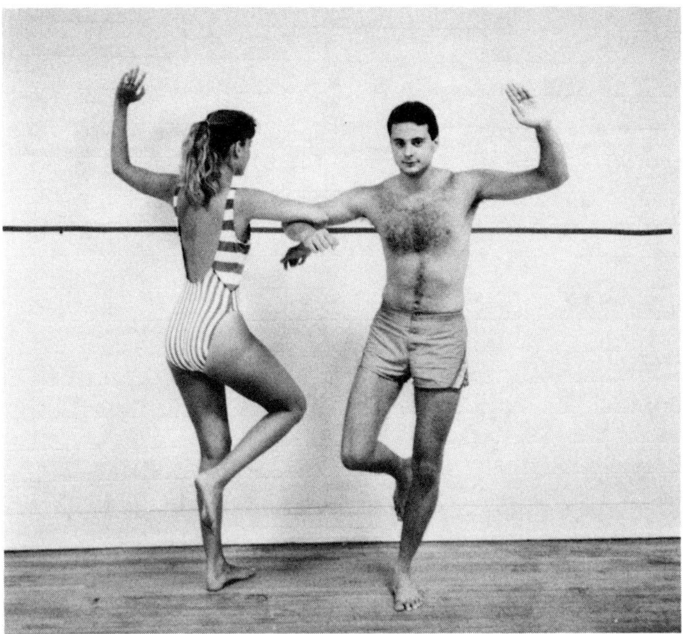

Muscle Groups

Hip Flexors, Iliopsoas, Gastrocnemius, Soleus, and Hamstrings.

Body Position

1. Stand in chest deep water.
2. Stand next to your partner but face the opposite direction.
3. Lock your right arm at the elbow with your partner's right arm at the elbow.
4. Raise your left arm high keeping it bent at the elbow.

Execution

1. Jog briskly around in a clockwise direction.
2. Change arms and circle in the opposite direction.

Key Points

1. Keep the leg lift high as you jog around.
2. Keep the body tall and in good alignment.
3. Move around briskly but be careful not to slip on the bottom of the pool.

Do-si-do

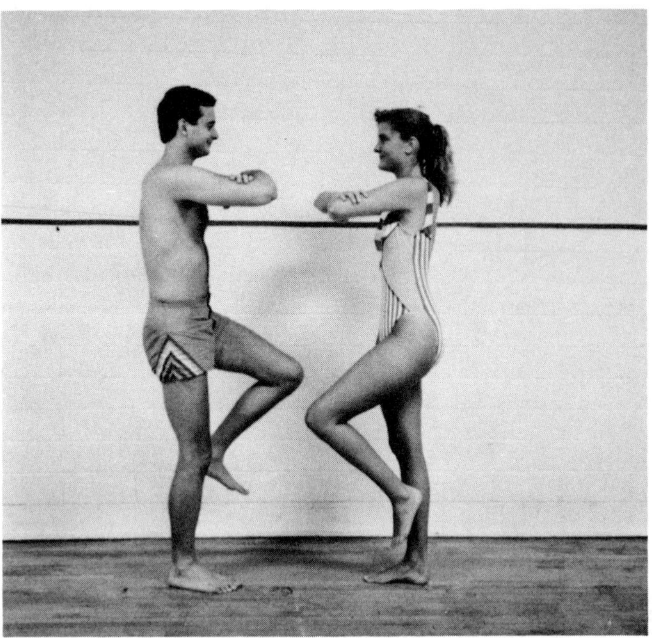

Muscle Groups

Hip Flexors and Extensors, Quadriceps, Gastrocnemius, Hamstrings, and Soleus.

Body Position

1. Stand in chest deep water.
2. Cross the arms at shoulder height with the hands placed on the opposite arm just above the elbow.

Execution

1. Start out facing your partner.
2. Circle clockwise around your partner, keeping the arm position high and above the water.
3. You will pass your partner face-to-face and back-to-back.
4. Change direction and repeat the motion.

Key Points

1. Keep the leg lift high as you jog around.
2. Keep the body tall and in good alignment.
3. Move around briskly, but be careful not to slip on the bottom of the pool.

Partner Carry

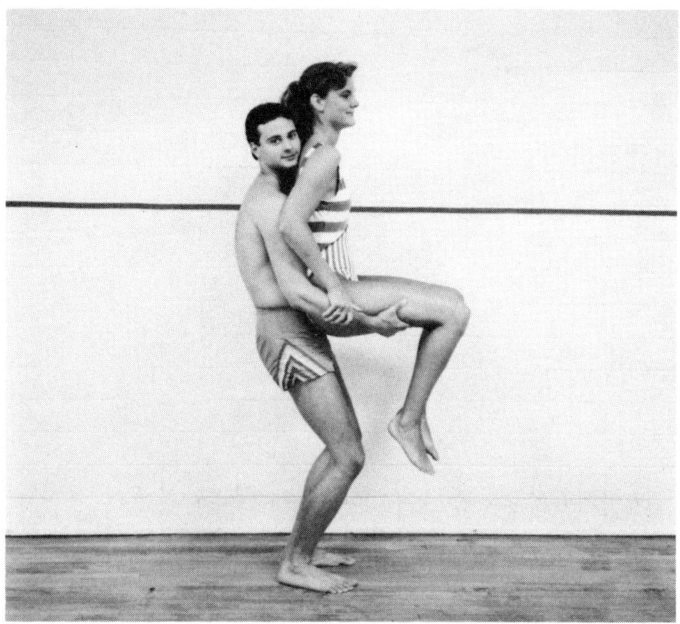

Muscle Groups

Biceps, Sacrospinalis, Hip Flexors and Hip Extensors.

Body Position

1. Make a seat with your hands at waist height.
2. Have your partner sit in the seat.
3. Hold your partner with the elbows slightly bent.

Execution

1. While holding your partner, push them to the other side of the pool.
2. After reaching the other side of the pool, change positions with your partner.
3. Push the original carrier back to the starting position.

Key Points

1. The carrier should keep the back straight.
2. Keep the body in good alignment as you push your partner.
3. Be careful not to slip on the bottom of the pool.

COOL-DOWN

7

The cool-down portion of the workout should allow the body to relax and the heart rate to return to its resting rate. This segment will include a variety of stretching exercises to assist in the elimination of exercise waste products (lactic acid) and to decrease the chance of muscle soreness and/or cramping.

During this time, you should breathe evenly and deeply. The heart rate will begin to drop as the body recovers from the aerobic exercise period. As mentioned previously, the recovery period will decrease as your cardiovascular fitness level improves. This is an indication that your heart is functioning at a more efficient level.

The cool-down will usually last from 5–10 minutes. Close and frequent checks of your heart rate will help determine when the body has cooled down sufficiently. Your heart rate should be below the target area when the cool-down is completed and close, if not at, your resting heart rate.

Bottom to Top

Calf Stretch

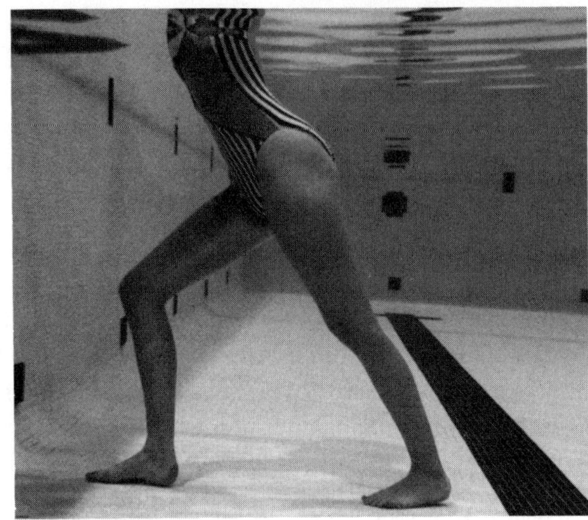

Muscle Groups

Gastrocnemius, and Soleus.

Body Position

1. Stand facing the side of the pool with the hands shoulder width apart and hold-ing on to the side.
2. Extend the right leg out behind with the foot flat on the bottom of the pool and the toes of the feet perpendicular to the side of the pool.
3. Place the left foot near the side of the pool with the toes perpendicular to the side of the pool.

Execution

1. Bend the left knee toward the side of the pool keeping the right foot flat on the bottom of the pool.
2. Bend the arms and lean the body toward the side of the pool.
3. Hold this position 6–10 seconds.
4. Repeat the sequence with the other leg.

Key Points

1. Keep both feet pointed toward the wall of the pool.
2. Keep the body straight and do not thrust the hip out.
3. Lean only until you feel the stretch, then hold the position.
4. Do not lock the knee of the extended leg.

Quadricep and Ankle Stretch

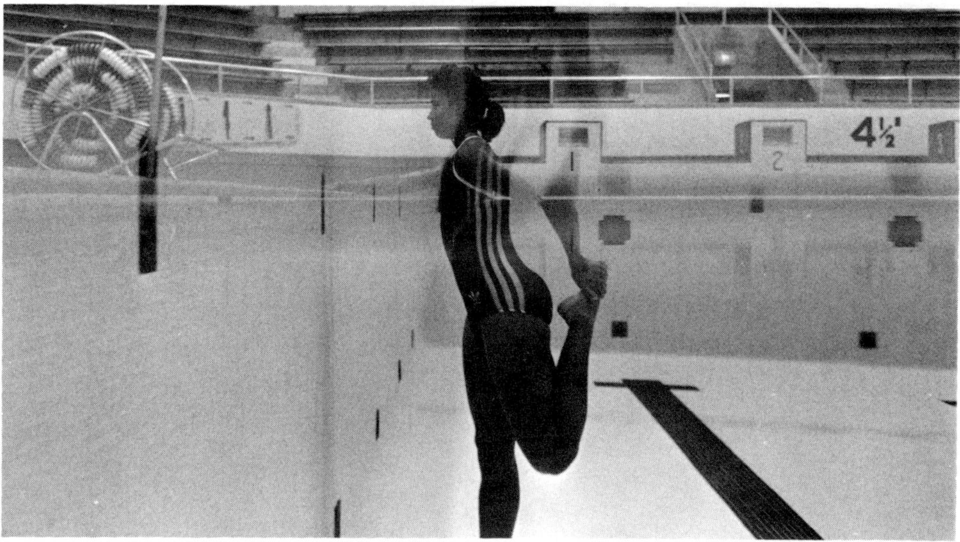

Muscle Groups

Quadriceps, Hip Flexors, and Tibialis Anterior.

Body Position

1. Stand facing the side of the pool with the hands shoulder width apart on the side of the pool.

Execution

1. Place the body weight on the right leg.
2. Bend the left leg up behind you and hold the toes with the left hand.
3. Pull the heel of the left foot to the buttocks.
4. Hold this position for 6–10 seconds.
5. Repeat the sequence with the left leg.

Key Points

1. Keep the body tall and the weight over the support leg.
2. Keep the knee of the bent leg pointed down toward the bottom of the pool.
3. Do not lock the knee of the support leg.

Leg Swing

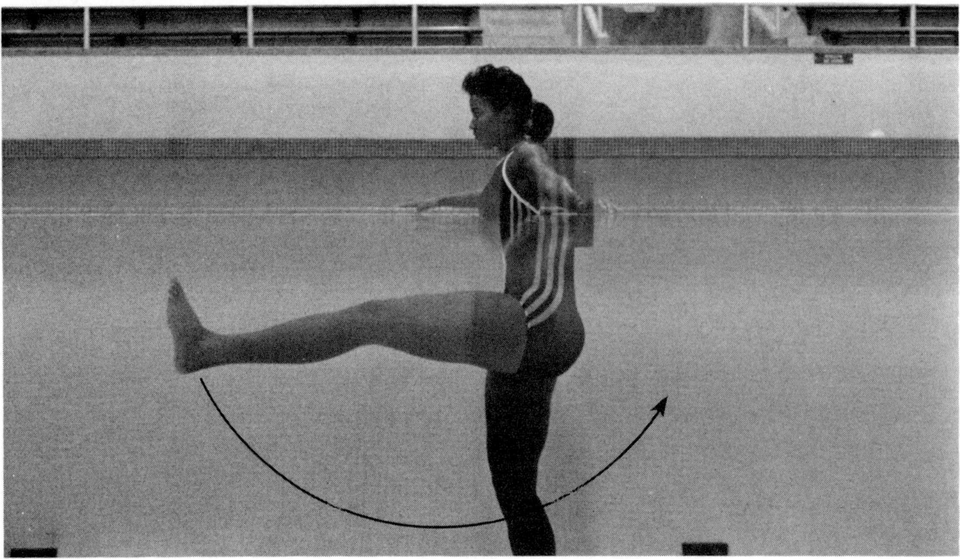

Muscle Groups

Hip Flexors and Hip Extensors.

Body Position

1. Stand with the left side to the pool wall and the left hand on the side of the pool.
2. Support your weight on the left leg.
3. Relax the foot of the right leg.

Execution

1. From the hip, lift the right leg comfortably up in front of the body.
2. Swing the right leg down by the left leg.
3. From the hip, lift the right leg comfortably up in back of the body.
4. Swing the right leg down by the left leg.
5. Repeat the sequence 8–15 times.
6. Change legs and repeat.

Key Points

1. Relax the hip, leg, and foot to create a comfortable, swinging motion.
2. Do not arch the back on the back-swing of the leg.
3. Keep the body tall and in good alignment.

Jello Shake

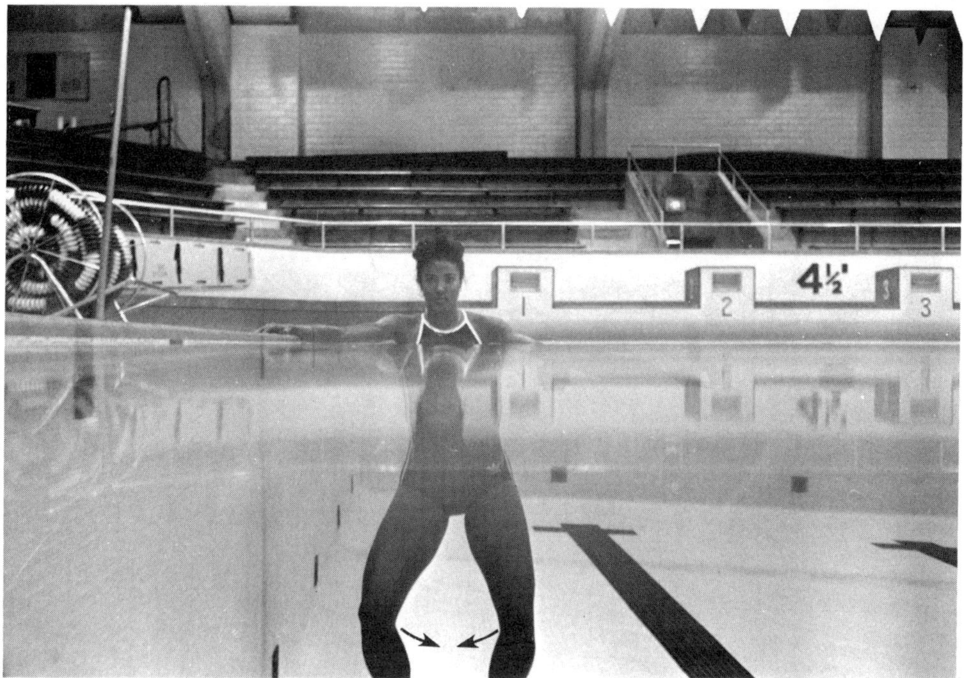

Muscle Groups

Quadriceps, Hip Adductors and Abductors.

Body Position

1. Step away from the side of the pool.
2. Separate the feet, placing them outside the width of the shoulders on the bottom of the pool.
3. Relax the legs and bend the knees slightly.

Execution

1. Shake the legs keeping the feet stationary.
2. Thighs and calves should move freely in the water.

Key Points

1. Bend only at the knees, not at the waist.
2. The more relaxed the legs are, the freer the muscle movement.

Straight Arm Shoulder Stretch

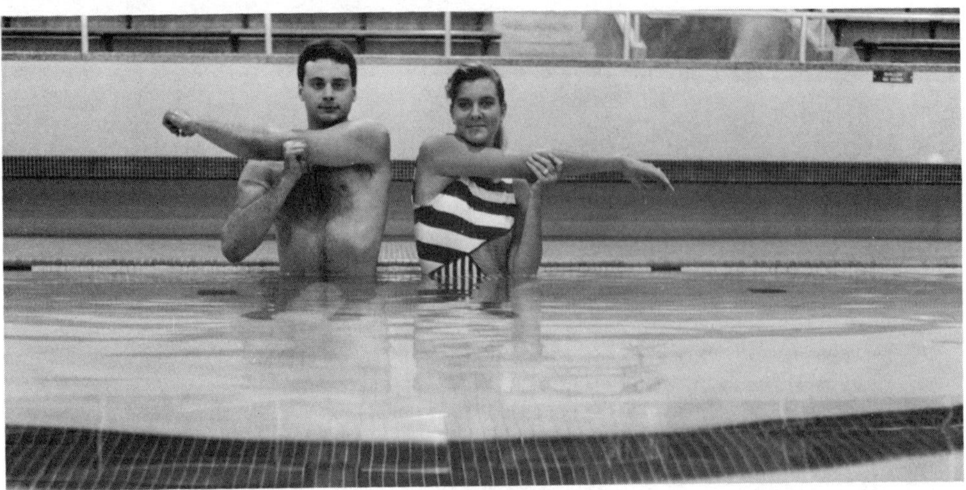

Muscle Groups

Posterior Deltoids, Rhomboids, and Latissimus Dorsi.

Body Position

1. Stand away from the side of the pool.
2. Separate the feet about shoulder width apart, keeping the body weight evenly distributed on both feet.

Execution

1. Place the right arm across in front of the body at shoulder height.
2. Hold the right arm above the elbow with the left hand.
3. Apply pressure with the left hand pulling the right arm close across the body and under the chin.
4. Hold the position for 6–10 seconds.
5. Repeat the motion with the other arm.

Key Points

1. Pressure should be constant.
2. Discomfort in the joint means you are pulling too hard.
3. You may experience greater flexibility in one shoulder.

Bent Arm Shoulder Stretch

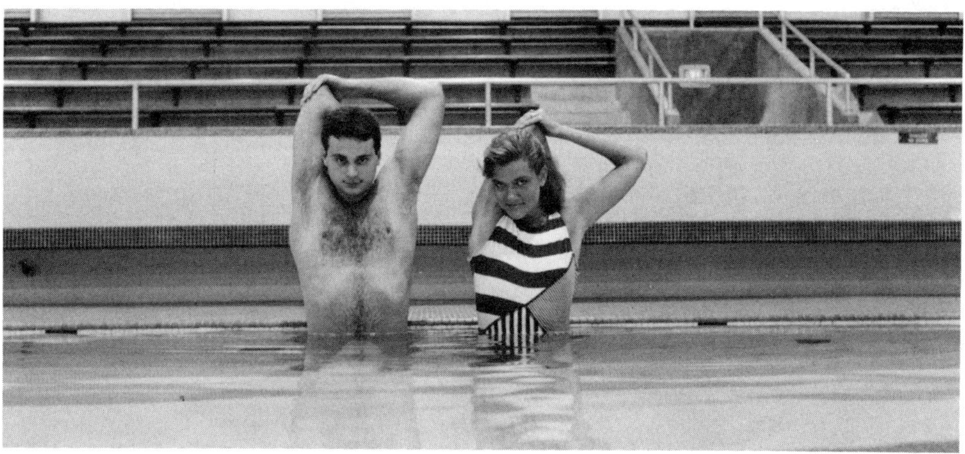

Muscle Groups

Deltoids and Serratus Anterior.

Body Position

1. Stand away from the side of the pool.
2. Separate the feet about shoulder width apart, keeping the body weight evenly distributed on both feet.

Execution

1. Place the right arm behind the head, allowing the elbow to bend and point up toward the ceiling or sky.
2. Take the left hand and place it just above the right elbow.
3. Apply pressure gently, easing the right elbow to the left.
4. Hold the position for 6–10 seconds.
5. Repeat the motion with the other arm.

Key Points

1. Keep the body tall and in good alignment.
2. Do not over stretch the arm and shoulder.
3. Relax the bent elbow.

Shoulder Shrug

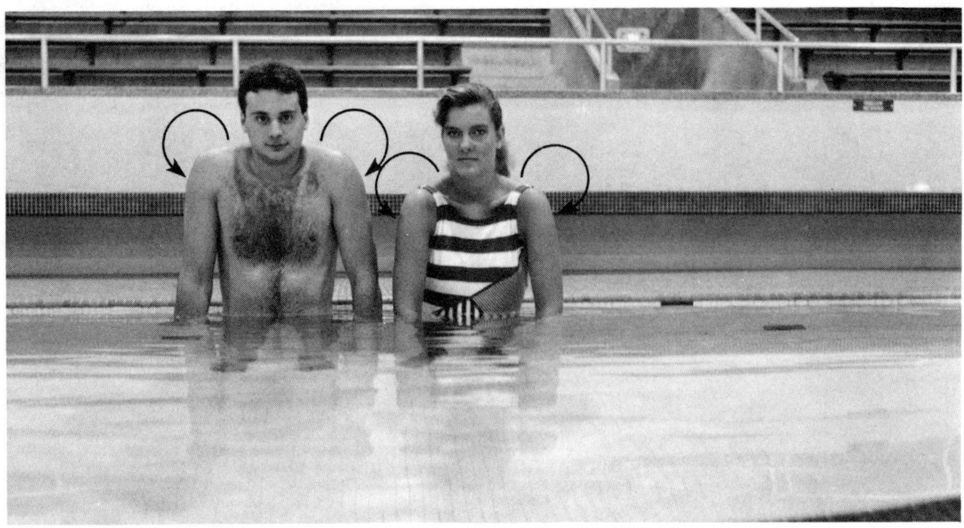

Muscle Groups

Trapezius.

Body Position

1. Stand away from the side of the pool.
2. Separate the feet about shoulder width apart keeping the weight evenly distributed on both feet.

Execution

1. Elevate both shoulders trying to "hug the ears."
2. Roll the shoulders forward.
3. Drop the shoulders down.
4. Roll the shoulders backward.
5. Repeat the motions several times in one direction and then change direction.

Key Points

1. Keep the shoulders as relaxed as possible.
2. Work through the full range of shoulder motion.
3. This exercise can also be done with the shoulders under the water.

Head Drop

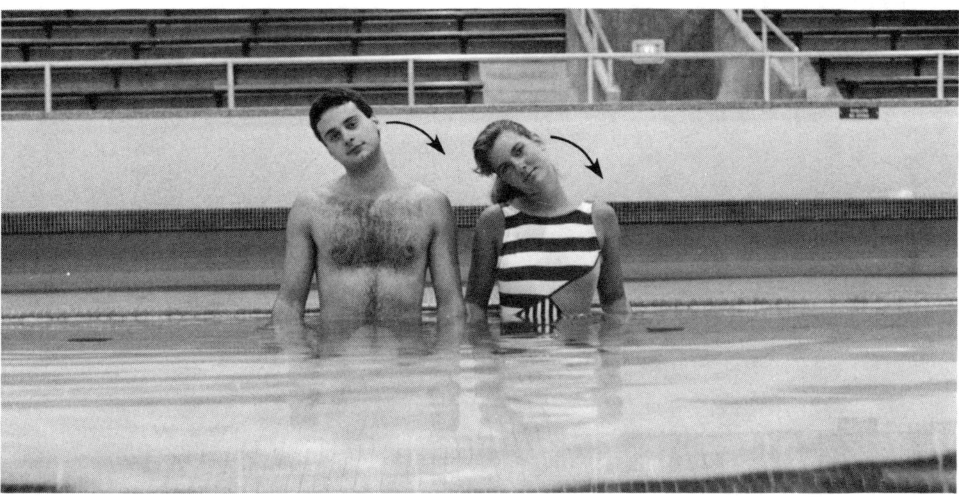

Muscle Groups

Sternocleidomastoid.

Body Position

1. Stand away from the side of the pool.
2. Separate the feet about shoulder width apart keeping the body weight evenly distributed on both feet.

Execution

1. Drop the head slowly to the right side.
2. Hold this position for 6–10 seconds.
3. Drop the head slowly to the left side.
4. Hold this position for 6–10 seconds.
5. Repeat the sequence several times to each side.

Key Points

1. Do not rotate the head from the neck.
2. Do not drop the head forward and back.
3. Keep the stretch static and comfortable.

A series of pre- and post-fitness screening tests will be administered to assess your present fitness level and the improvement you have made by the end of the semester. The results of these tests will enable you to evaluate your level of fitness and areas needing further improvement. By using the results of the fitness screening tests, a water aerobics program can be more accurately designed to fit your fitness needs and fitness goals.

In-Water Jog

An *In-Water Jog* test will be used to help in assessing your present cardiovascular endurance. This is a sub-maximal test of cardiovascular endurance, so, you should have no difficulty completing the test.

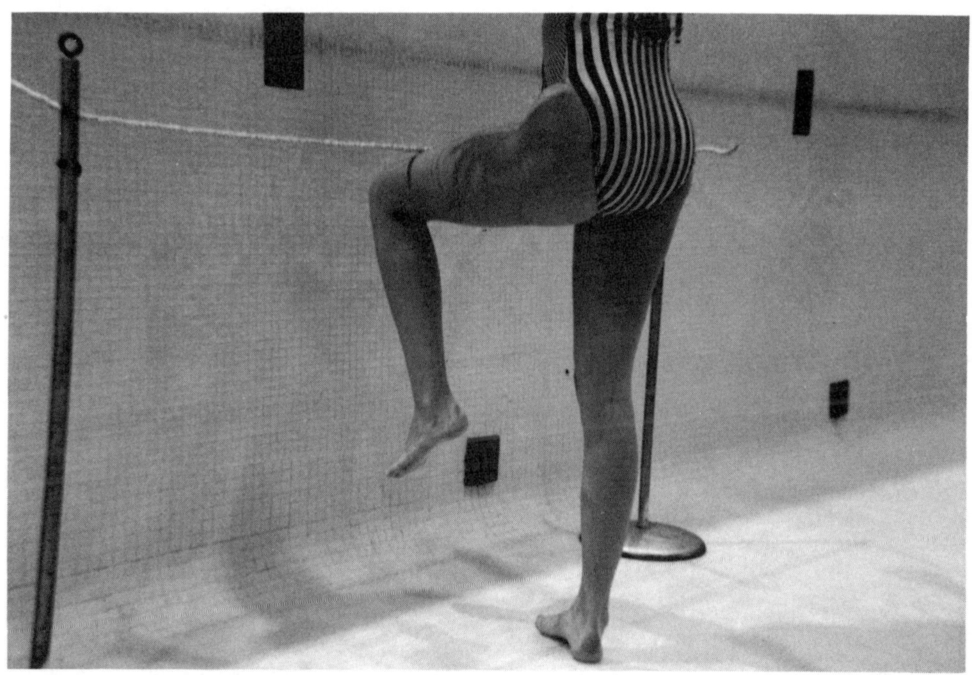

Stand in chest deep water facing the side of the pool and at least an arm's length away from the side of the pool. A rope will be stretched between three submerged support standards. The standards will be placed parallel to and three feet from the side of the pool. The height of the rope will be graduated starting from a low point at the shallow end of the pool and reaching its highest point at the deeper end of the pool. Your position along the rope will be determined by your height. When lifting your leg in a jogging motion, the rope should just touch the middle of the quadricep when the hip joint is at a 90 degree angle to the leg. The knee should also be bent at a 90 degree angle. The rope is used as the reference point for the bent-leg elevation during the jogging motion.

The test lasts three minutes with an audio cassette tape maintaining the cadence for you. The beat will be the cue for you to change legs in the jogging motion. Be sure to keep up the pace of the jogging motion in accordance with the voice commands on the tape! If you go too slowly or too fast, the accuracy of the test results will be adversely affected. The tempo of the test is brisk 156 beats per minute.

At the conclusion of the test, you will be asked to turn around with your back to the pool and find your radial (wrist) pulse. Two other students will be asked to assist in the pulse count by finding the right and left carotid pulse. Ten seconds have been allotted in which to find these three pulse points. The tape will then instruct you and your partners to take the pulse for a 15-second count. This first count is considered your exercise pulse. The pulse taking will be repeated two more times at the one- and two-minute time intervals. The second count is the recovery rate. This pulse count will be used to determine your starting cardiovascular fitness level and your improvement at the end of the semester. As your cardiovascular fitness improves, the second or +1 pulse count will drop. This is an indication that the heart and circulatory system are functioning more efficiently.

Crunch and Front Dip

A *Crunch* test will be used to determine your abdominal strength and endurance. The test will last for one minute during which time you will be asked to do as many crunches as possible. A partner will count the number of crunches performed and check for proper body position and execution of the crunch.

To begin, you will lie on the floor with your legs bent at the knee and your feet flat on the floor and close to the buttocks. Cross your arms over the chest and grasp the shoulders with your hands. The arms and hands must remain in this position throughout the testing period. If the hands come off the shoulders, the crunch will not count.

Contract the abdominal muscles and roll the upper body toward the legs, allowing the shoulders to come off of the floor. The lower back and hips should remain in contact with the floor. Return to the original starting position and repeat the motion until the one-minute test period is over or muscle fatigue occurs to prevent continuation. Make sure to maintain tight, contracted abdominal muscles during the test and to breath evenly and deeply.

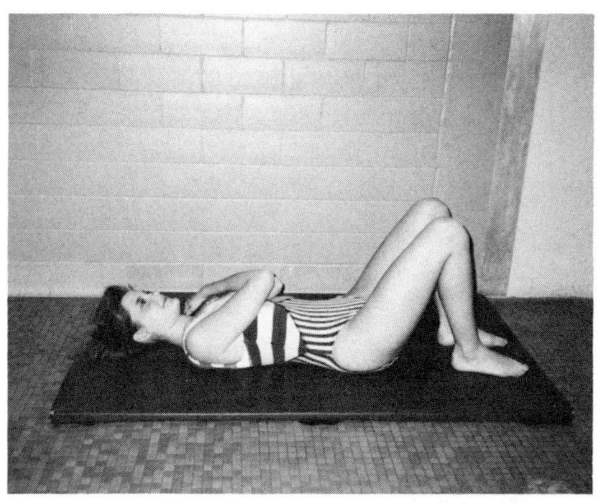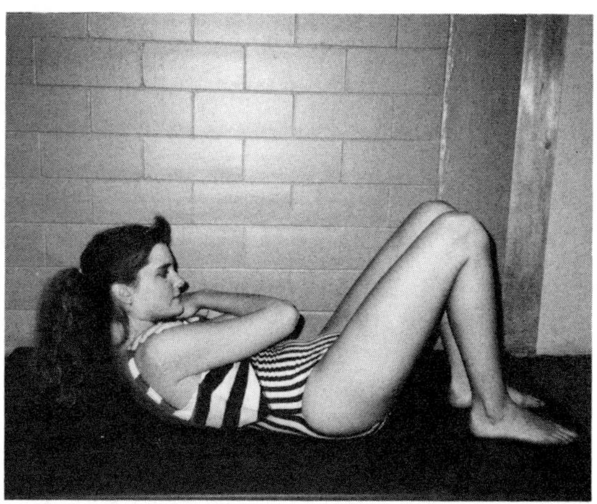

Shoulder girdle strength and endurance will be assessed through the use of the *Front Dip*. This test item has already been explained in Chapter V under warm-up exercises and visual demonstrations are shown in photos on page 38. As in the crunch test, you will have one minute to perform as many front dips as you can. You will start with your hands on the side of the pool just outside the width of the shoulders. The water level should be at chest depth. Push up to a straight arm position. Each time you dip down achieving a 90 degree angle at the elbow and return to a straight arm position will count as one repetition. The dip will not count if you kick your feet, push off from the bottom of the pool or fail to achieve the required 90 degree angle at the elbow. Repeat the motion until the one- minute time period has expired or until muscle fatigue occurs, and no more dips can be performed. Breathe evenly and deeply during the test and always do as many dips as possible so an accurate accounting of shoulder strength and endurance can be taken.

Sit-and-Reach

Flexibility will be assessed through the use of a *Sit-and-Reach* test. A wooden box and yardstick will be used to administer this test.

Sit on the floor with your back and buttocks flat against the wall and your legs extended straight out in front. Place your feet against the end of the wooden box. With the shoulders flat against the wall, extend your arms out in front and parallel with your legs. The yardstick on top of the box will be adjusted so the end is at the tips of your fingers. Moving the yardstick to the fingers will take into consideration individual variations in arm and leg length.

Bending forward from the hips, slide forward with the hands along the yardstick as far as you can. Hold the stretch at the furthest point so a reading can be taken from the yardstick. Do not bounce into the stretch. Keep the legs straight, but do not lock them at the knees.

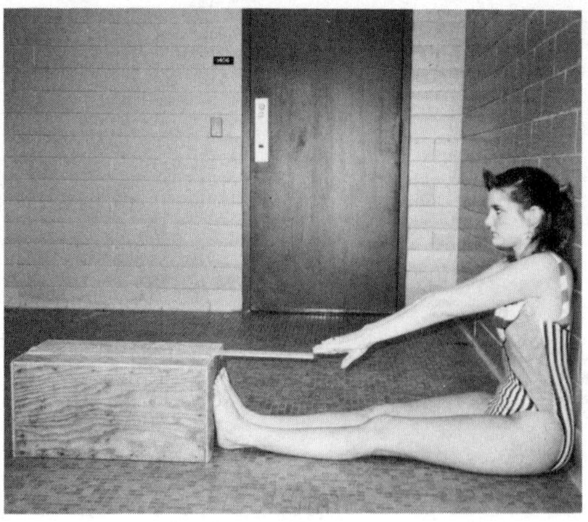

This test will help determine lower back flexibility. At the end of the semester, improvement in this area of fitness should be quite evident.

At the completion of these tests, an assessment of your fitness level will be made by your instructor. This fitness assessment will enable you to realistically set up your fitness goals for the semester, and ultimately set goals for future fitness programs.

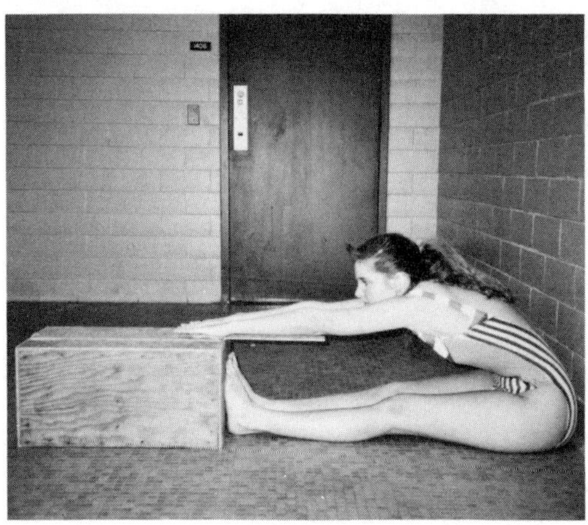

REFERENCES

Adams, Ronald C. and Daniel, Alfred N. and McCabbin, Jeffrey A. and Rullman, Lee. *Games, Sports and Exercise for the Physically Handicapped.* Philadelphia: Lee and Febiger, 1972.

Allard, Kevyn. "Water Workout: Cool in The Pool." *Women's Sports and Fitness.* Vol. 9, August, 1987.

Bayne, Cheryl. "Water Aerobics—The Exercise Wave of the Future!" *Parks and Recreation.* February, 1987.

Brown, H. Larry. *Lifetime Fitness.* Scottsdale, Arizona: Gorsuch Scarisbrick, Publishers, 1986.

Cooper, Kenneth H. *The Aerobics Program For Total Well-Being.* New York: M-Evans and Company, Inc., 1982.

Eichstaedt, Carl B. and Kalakian, Leonard H. *Developmental/Adapted Physical Education.* New York: MacMillan Publishing Company, 1987.

Evenbeck, Betty. "Aquatic Exercise Taking Shape." *Journal of Physical Education, Recreation, and Dance.* October, 1986.

Fox, Sir Cyril S. *Water.* 15 E. 40th Street, N.Y., 16, New York: The Philosophical Library, Inc., 1952.

France, Kenneth. *Body Conditioning—The Thinking Person's Guide To Aerobic Fitness.* Atlanta, Georgia: Humanics New Age, 1985.

Gajda, R. and Dominquez, R. *Total Body Training.* Warner Books, Inc., 1982.

Haslam, Robert H.A.(M.D.) and Vallehitti, Peter J. (Ed.D). *Medical Problems in The Classroom.* Baltimore: University Park Press, 1975.

Jeppesen. *Open Water Sport Diver Manual.* 55 Inverness Drive, East, Englewood, Colorado: Jeppesen Sanderson, Inc., 1986.

Katz, Jane. *The W.E.T. Workout.* New York, N.Y.: Facts On File Publications, 1985.

King, Thomas. *Water.* New York: MacMillian Company, 1953.

Koszuta, Laurie Einstein. "Water Exercise Causes Ripples." *The Physician and Sports Medicine.* Vol. 14, No. 10, October, 1986.

Krasevec, Joseph A. and Grimes, Diane C. *HydroRobics.* P.O. Box 3, West Point, N.Y., 10996: Leisure Press, 1985.

Mannerber, M.D. and Roth, Don and June. *Aerobic Nutrition.* 2 Park Avenue, New York, N.Y.: Elsevier-Dutton Publishing Company, Inc., 1981.

Nieman, D.C. *The Sports Medicine Fitness Course.* Bull Publishing Company, 1986.

Payne, Wayne A. and Hahn, Dale B. *Understanding Your Health.* 11803 Westline Industrial Drive, St. Louis, Missouri, 63146: Mirror/Mosby Publishing, 1989.

Seaman, Janet A. and DePauw, Karen P. *The New Adapted Physical Education—A Developmental Approach.* Mayfield Publishing Company, 1982.

Sova, R. ''A Workout That's All Wet.'' *Dance Exercise Today*. Vol. 5, May, 1987.

The American Red Cross. *Adapted Aquatics*. Garden City, N.J.: Doubleday Company, Inc. 1977.

Thompson, Terri L. ''Aerobics—Water Workouts.'' *Dance Teacher Now*. Vol. 9, July/August, 1987.

"Using Your Heart Rate As A Guide To Your Exercise Level.'' *The Health Letter*. Volume XVII, No. 9, May 8, 1981.

White, Sue W. ''Something New for The Pool.'' *Journal of Physical Education, Recreation, and Dance*. February, 1984.

APPENDIX A

Training/Target Heart Rate

Name ____

Age_________________

Resting Heart Rate (1 Minute Count):

(A)______________ (B)______________ (C)_______________

Karvonen Formula:	A	B	C	D
Max. Working Heart				
Rate (220-Age)	______	______	______	______
Subtract Resting	______	______	______	______
Heart Rate	______	______	______	______
Heart Rate Reserve	______	______	______	______
Multiply % of	______	______	______	______
Working Capacity	x .6______	x .7______	x .8______	x .9______
Answer	______	______	______	______
Add Resting HR	______	______	______	______
Target Heart Rate	______	______	______	______
6 Second Range	______	______	______	______

APPENDIX B

Fitness Screening

Name____Hour_________Day________

       Last   First   Middle

Age ________Sex________ ID#________-________-________ Ht.________Wt.______

Screening Tests

Crunch: Entrance _____________   Exit__________________

Front Dips: Entrance _____________   Exit__________________

Flexibility: Entrance _____________   Exit__________________

In-Water Jog:

Entrance	EOT	+1	+2
Counter 1			
Counter 2			
Testee			
Avg. C1 & C2			
Exit	EOT	+1	+2
Counter 1			
Counter 2			
Testee			
Avg. C1 & C2			

Appendix C

Muscular Anatomy: Front View

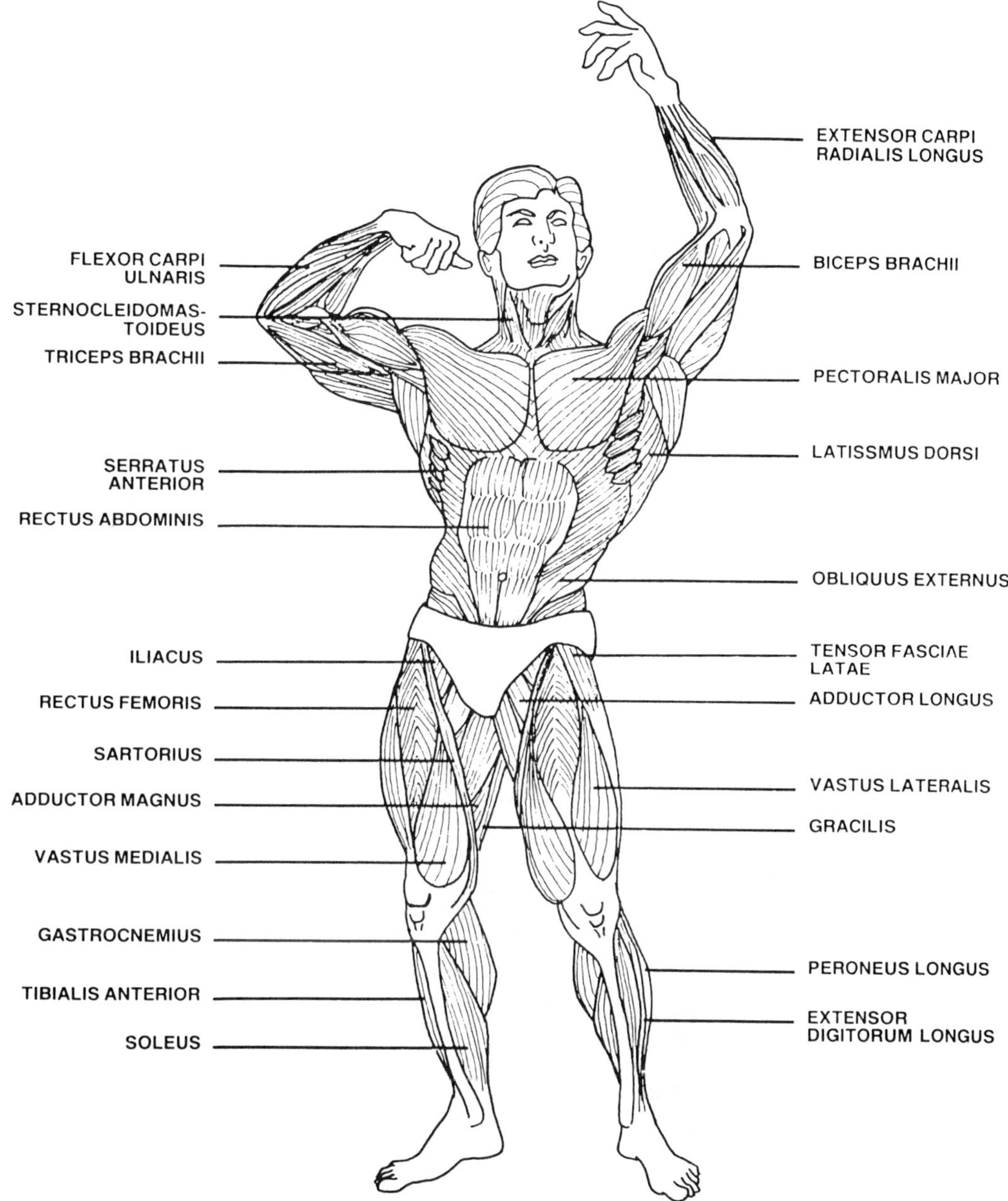

Muscular Anatomy: Back View

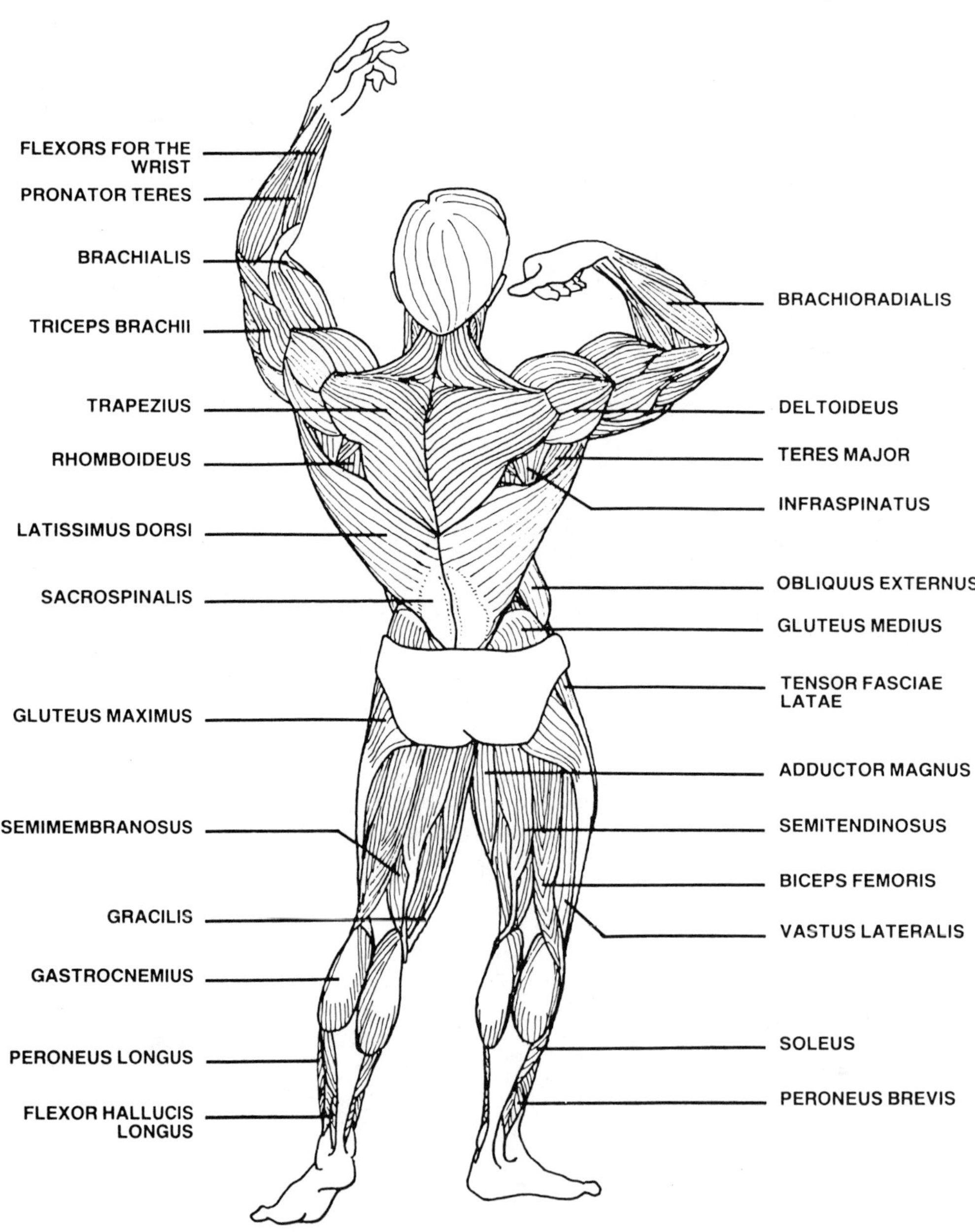

Printed with permission of Hydra-Fitness Industries, P.O. Box 599, Belton, Texas, 76513